A

PARENT'S

GUIDE TO

ASTHMA

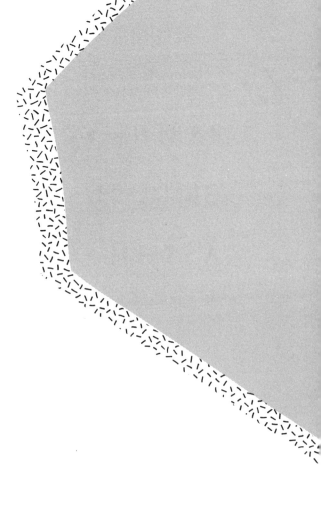

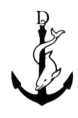

Doubleday

NEW YORK

LONDON

TORONTO

SYDNEY

AUCKLAND

A PARENT'S GUIDE TO ASTHMA

NANCY SANDER

Published by Doubleday, a division of
Bantam Doubleday Dell Publishing Group, Inc.
666 Fifth Avenue, New York, New York 10103

Doubleday and the portrayal of an anchor with a
dolphin are trademarks of Doubleday, a division
of Bantam Doubleday Dell Publishing Group, Inc.

Library of Congress Cataloging-in-Publication Data

Sander, Nancy.
 A parent's guide to asthma.

 Bibliography: p.
 Includes index.
 1. Asthma in children—Popular works. I. Title.
RJ436.A8S26 1989 618.92′238 88-25682
ISBN 0-385-24478-9

DESIGNED BY—DIANE STEVENSON/SNAP-HAUS GRAPHICS

DEDICATION

WITHOUT THE SUPPORT OF MY LOVING FAMILY THIS BOOK would not be a reality. Nor would I ever have seen the need to write this book without experiencing the fear and loneliness of parenting a child with severe asthma. So I dedicate this book with love to my daughter, Brooke Daylen Sander, who has taught me many things, and, from the looks of it, will continue to do so for the remainder of my days; to my husband, Dale, who loves me enough to have made it possible for me to write this book; to my sons Michael and Daniel, who washed dishes, vacuumed, and took care of Brooke and Joseph as needed without *too* much complaint; and to Joseph, my youngest son, whose quiet, refreshing hugs are always welcome.

CONTENTS

PREFACE   xiii

FOREWORD   xv

INTRODUCTION   xix

PART I GETTING ASTHMA UNDER CONTROL

1 OUR STORY   3

2 ASTHMA BASICS   19

       Triggers—According to Plan—Early
       Warning Signals—Keeping a Diary

3 MYTHS AND OLD WIVES' TALES   36

       Myth #1: It's All in Your Head   37
       Myth #2: Asthma Is the Result of a
                  Poor Mother and Child
                  Relationship   40
       Myth #3: Children Grow Out of
                  Asthma   42
       Myth #4: Move to Arizona   44
       Myth #5: Pet a Chihuahua   45
       Myth #6: Asthma Doesn't Kill Anyone
                  Anymore   46
       Myth #7: Asthma Doesn't Require
                  Medical Treatment   48
       Myth #8: Asthma Isn't Serious
                  Anymore   49

4 HOW TO FIND A GOOD DOCTOR   50

Quackery—Office Visit Form—Paying for
Health Care

5 WHAT PARENTS NEED TO KNOW ABOUT
MEDICATIONS, ALLERGY TESTS AND
IMMUNOTHERAPY   73

Inside the Medicine Cabinet—Medication
Myths—Therapies on the Horizon—How to
Help Your Child Learn to Swallow Pills
and Take Otherwise Foul-Tasting Medicines
—Allergy Testing—Preparing Your Child
for Allergy Testing and Immunotherapy—
Other Tests

6 TOOLS OF THE TRADE   105

Stethoscopes—Peak Flow Meters—
Nebulizers—Inhalers—Spacers—Other
Tools

7 ALLERGY-PROOFING YOUR HOME   126

Tackling the Bedroom—Air Filters—
Vacuums—Stop Smoking—Wood and Coal
Stoves—Pets—Food Allergies—Here Are
Some Tips for Parents with Kids on a
Different Diet from the Rest of the Family

—Milk—Sulfites—Soy—Living with the
Food-Allergic Child

P A R T   I I   **GROWING UP WITH ASTHMA**

8 FROM DIAPERS TO DATING   163

Birth to Age Two—Ages Three to Six—Ages
Seven to Twelve—Teens—At Every Age

9 ASTHMA GOES TO SCHOOL   202

Your Child's Teacher—Getting Ready to
Start School—Allergies at School—Physical
Education—Should My Child Stay Home
Today?—The Effect of Theophylline on
Learning and School Behavior—Be a
Volunteer—Making Up Is Not So Hard to
Do

10 SPORTS AND OUTDOOR ADVENTURES   218

Sports—Camp Mini-Wheeze-No-More—
Family Camping—Scouting

11 PLANNING A FAMILY VACATION   231

Vacation-Planning Checklist—Packing List
—Other Tips

12 ASTHMA IS A FAMILY AFFAIR   244

Sibling Rivalry—Marriage and Divorce—
Single-Parenting the Asthmatic Child—Part-
time Single Parenting—When Both Parents
Work

AFTERWORD: LOOKING FORWARD   261

RESOURCES   265

Books and Pamphlets—Food Allergies—
Newsletters—Videos—Products—Support
Groups—Organizations—Medical Journals
—Treatment Centers and Hospitals—
Asthma and Allergic Disease Centers—
Centers for Interdisciplinary Research on
Immunologic Diseases—Scholarships—
Asthma Camps

INDEX   291

ACKNOWLEDGMENTS

I WOULD LIKE TO THANK DR. MARTHA VETTER WHITE, NOT only for her part as medical editor of this book, but also for our asthma management plan. It works! Thanks also to Debbie Scherrer, my good friend and the mother of two children with asthma, who jumped through hoops to keep things running smoothly at Mothers of Asthmatics, Inc., while I was writing and who also contributed several of the stories. Debbie even read this book almost as many times as I rewrote it! A special thanks to Allan M. Weinstein, M.D., author of *Asthma: The Complete Guide,* for his inspiration and guidance, and for writing the Foreword to this book. And to Kathy Sickels, my talented artist friend, I give many thanks for her graphic illustrations in this book.

Thanks also to Jackie, Sidney, Memo, John Maddox, Moises, Nancy, Janice, Bob, and Linda, and to the many parents who have shared their stories in this book.

PREFACE

PHYSICIANS COMMONLY PRESCRIBE THE MEDICATIONS DIS-cussed in this book for asthmatics of all ages. Some are prescribed more often for children while others are prescribed more frequently for adults.

Many parents may have noticed that their children with asthma have been prescribed medications that had received Food and Drug Administration (FDA) approval only for persons twelve years and older. Surprisingly, many if not most medications on the market do not have FDA approval for use by pregnant females or for children below twelve years of age. The reason for this is primarily economic: obtaining FDA approval for children requires additional clinical trials employing the drug in children, and this is costly. The lack of FDA approval for children under twelve does not mean that the drug is unsafe or ineffective. It simply means that safety and efficacy for children have not been established according to FDA guidelines. Once a drug has received FDA approval for any indication, physicians may use their best medical judgment in prescribing the medication for age groups or disease categories for which the drug has not received FDA approval. Thus it is not unusual for medications (for example, albuterol [Proventil, Ventolin] inhalers) to be prescribed for children under twelve even though they have FDA approval only for patients twelve and over.

A Parent's Guide to Asthma contains current practical information about the medications available for people with asthma—regardless of whether they have FDA approval for children under twelve or under six. This book does not intend to comment on the appropriateness of prescribing medications for age groups not covered by the FDA approval. Instead, this book will provide information about the medications your doctor has to choose from. It is the responsibility of your doctor to determine the best medication or combination of medications for your child.

Martha V. White, M.D.
National Institutes of Health
Bethesda, Maryland

FOREWORD

WITH NANCY SANDER ON YOUR SIDE, YOU ARE NOT ALONE. Her energy is contagious—encouraging parents to learn more about asthma, a serious yet manageable illness. She knows firsthand what it is like to have a child with difficult asthma. Her own frustrations in coping with her daughter, Brooke's, asthma prompted her to take action. She sought out expert advice and read extensively. One result, the fund of helpful information in her newsletter, *MA Report*, has prompted some to dub her the "Ann Landers of asthma and allergy."

Asthma is a leading cause of illness, affecting up to 10 percent of America's children and accounting for up to 20 percent of missed school days. Asthma is the most common reason children are admitted to most pediatric hospitals, with the hospitalization rate for children up 225 percent since 1969 (up 67 percent for adults). Of greatest concern, the death rate from asthma is on the rise in spite of the fact that asthma, as a rule, is a manageable, reversible illness. Unfortunately, we do not know the cause for this increased death rate. Studies being conducted under the direction of the American Academy of Allergy and Immunology and the National Institutes of Health cover a range of factors—environmental and industrial pollutants, allergen exposure, food additives, and aspirin sensitivity, as well as the emotional state of the individual. Attention also now focuses on the fact that asthma often is not regarded as a serious illness, an attitude that often results in undertreatment or delay in seeking treatment, with patients relying on the emergency room for asthma care.

Even though some of these factors may be beyond one's control, one must remember that although asthma cannot be cured, it can be well managed. Successful management of asthma requires patient education.

I have learned from my patients that they want as much information as possible about asthma care. Asthma can be frustrating and difficult to understand. An array of factors triggers symptoms and a variety of techniques apply for proper use of each medication. Understanding and organizing this information is the key to working most effectively with one's doctor to tailor an asthma self-management plan.

A Parent's Guide to Asthma emphasizes the practical aspects of day-to-day asthma management. The book contains a wealth of clearly presented, well-organized information about dealing with asthma in a myriad of settings—in school, at home, on vacation, during sports, and at camp. The book's suggestions for effective coordination and communication with the child's doctor will make it possible for any parent to be part of the asthma management team. It presents the proper uses of asthma management "tools," including nebulizers, peak flow meters and spacing devices. And Nancy Sander also looks at asthma from a chronological perspective, offering insight into the ability of each age group to use these tools. Every parent will find invaluable the book's resource guide, which lists addresses and phone numbers for the full range of asthma and allergy services—everything from alergy-free products for the home to asthma-oriented camps and support groups.

Nancy Sander's insights into the impact of asthma on family life draw not only from personal experience but from her newsletter readership as well. Clearly there is no one more capable than she to present this long overdue perspective.

A Parent's Guide to Asthma will comfort you, reassure you that others share your challenges, and guide you toward successful asthma care. I heartily applaud Nancy Sander's contribution to asthma education and this, her latest effort.

Allan Weinstein, M.D.
Washington, D.C.

INTRODUCTION

I SPENT SIX LONELY, FRUSTRATING, AND FRIGHTENING YEARS
fighting to help my daughter breathe. Brooke has asthma and
allergies. Then I discovered the freedom of asthma under
control, and I decided to share the great news with others. I
founded a nonprofit organization called Mothers of Asthmatics, Inc., which included a "support system in a newsletter"
called *MA Report.* The organization, which began as a simple
newsletter in November of 1985, has grown and grown, and
had six thousand members in 1988.

Once, even to hope that Brooke would ever be free of
asthma's clutches was almost too much to dream. But when
it did happen, it was the end of countless asthma-related hospitalizations, emergency room visits, and even unscheduled
office visits. It was the beginning of a regular life un-
hampered by asthma.

But it didn't happen by accident or by a secret miracle process. The solution was lots of hard work, a willingness to
learn, and working with the right doctors. What happened to
us can happen to you. I hope this book will help you dupli-
cate our success. However, I must warn you that the management plan that worked for Brooke may not be the *exact* plan
that will work for your child. Like a fingerprint, asthma is
unique in each person. It will be your goal to work with your

doctor to develop an asthma management plan tailored for your child.

It *can* be done! *You are not alone.* There are millions of us around the world rocking our choking babies, giving breathing treatments, reading food labels, and sitting in doctors' offices. You will hear from some of those parents throughout this book as they share their frustrations and *victories.*

A Parent's Guide to Asthma will help you deal with the practical aspects of living with and raising a child with asthma. Though basic asthma education is presented throughout, **this is not a book on the medical management of asthma and allergies.** Let me immediately refer you to my favorite book on that subject, *Asthma: The Complete Guide to Self-Management of Asthma and Allergies for Patients and Their Families* by Dr. Allan M. Weinstein.

We will specifically address the needs of the child with asthma, his parents, and family during the most difficult period, between diagnosis and control. Asthma out of control, be it mild or severe, in infants or in older children, is a living nightmare. The more we as parents understand asthma, the less we fear it. The less we fear asthma, the more capable managers we become and the better able we are to help our children. This book will become your guide to controlling asthma's destructive force in your home.

This distressing period of adjustment will pass. As you understand asthma better and learn to recognize the early warning signals and triggers, you will begin to respond to them appropriately and life will stabilize. Asthma will interrupt your life less frequently. When you, too, can say that asthma no longer controls your life, won't you share this comfort with others? Though the hardships of the moment may be oppressive, the rewards of perseverance will endure. May God bless you as you read this book.

GETTING ASTHMA UNDER CONTROL

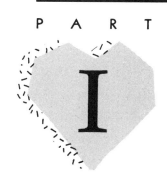

I

OUR STORY

"**H**URRY! THE BABY *IS* COMING!" I INsisted. The nurse had examined me moments before and declared me far from ready to be taken into delivery. Dale looked up and down the hallway. "Hurry, please hurry!" I pleaded. Somewhat reluctantly, he retrieved Dr. Fruiterman from the doctor's lounge.

"Dr. Fruiterman, the baby is coming," I said as he lifted the sheet. "You're right!" he said quickly. "Ready for a ride?" He hollered for a nurse as he and Dale maneuvered the labor bed into the hall in the direction of delivery room.

Minutes later I met my daughter, all nine pounds of her. With the miseries of labor and delivery behind me, I was in heaven and Dale was in love. Little did we know we had just given birth to a baby with an invisible time bomb—an infant with severe asthma and allergies.

Each feeding, Brooke nursed greedily before snoozing at my breast. But no sooner would I begin resting in the joy of my blessing than her little tummy would lurch and reverse her meal. "This baby is a spitter," I told Becky, my hospital roommate. Becky was having nursing problems of her own. Becky's supply of milk was overwhelming and my supply was being rejected. "Well, maybe things will be better when we get home."

Homecoming day, I dressed Brooke in a dainty pink and white dress with matching bonnet and booties, a gift from her doting aunt Jeanette. Becky leaned over the bassinet and cooed, "Poor baby, your momma thinks you are a baby doll that she can dress in frilly clothes and parade around." We both chuckled. Brooke was my princess, and I reasoned, after having two sons before her, that I was going to enjoy every moment of having a daughter.

Dale arrived to take us home. But when I picked Brooke up, her stomach lurched once again and she spit up all over me and her pink frillies. "Serves you right," Becky chided. We laughed. Had we known then what we know now, it would not have been laughter coming from that room.

Brooke continued to spit up what seemed to be every bit of milk she nursed. I'm not talking about normal baby dribbles, either. Brooke spit up in ounces and got it everywhere. I conscientiously ate nutritious meals including milk, eggs, and whole grains (the very foods to which she is most allergic, we were to later learn). I took my prenatal vitamins. Dale's mom was helping with the kids and house so I got plenty of rest. I was doing everything I could to make strong, nutritious milk, and this baby did nothing but throw it up.

Brooke lost weight and looked so thin and frail, you could see where the bones of her skull met. We tried various formulas, each with the same result as the breast milk. She was tested for digestive problems. Negative. Finally, we tried a feeding procedure the doctor said he and his colleague believed might help Brooke gain weight. We cooked Cream of Rice cereal into a thick paste, thinned it slightly with breast milk and fed Brooke while she was propped in her infant seat. Afterward, I nursed her and then returned her to the infant seat where she was to remain propped for thirty minutes. Brooke began to gain weight. Though she still vomited following each meal, enough of the food was staying down to nourish her.

Brooke, my skinny little princess, was quite unaware of her royal papers. Her face was peppered with pimples and rashes and often hives. Her skin was dry and rough. I didn't know the names to attach to her troubles, names like allergies, eczema and asthma. In 1978, the popular school of thought believed food allergies, and asthma in infants was virtually nonexistent; breast milk was considered customized health food. Symptoms were described as "things she will grow out of in a few months."

When Brooke was less than nine months old, her doctor left our health plan and we started seeing Dr. Cheryl McGee. After a few sick visits, prescriptions, creams, ear infections, fits of coughing and wheezing, Dr. McGee concluded, "Mrs. Sander, I think what we are dealing with here is asthma and allergies."

I had no idea what asthma was, so she explained that

asthma is a narrowing of the airways, which obstructs breathing. She said it could be controlled but Brooke was so young and her airways so small, we would have to monitor her asthma carefully.

Usually, parents remember a baby's first smile, step or word. But Brooke's life seemed to be made up of one attack or crisis after another, blurring the occasions of those firsts. Brooke's asthma persisted relentlessly. Night and day seemed to blend into each other.

When she was just shy of eighteen months old, we visited an allergist for evaluation. Part of this procedure included skin tests for allergies. The allergist pricked the skin on her back with needles and dropped an antigen (a concentrated substance to which the child is suspected of being allergic) on each prick site. He used a device which delivered ten pricks at once, and she was tested for forty items at each of two testing sessions.

To prepare Brooke as well as I could, considering her age, I explained that the allergy testing would not feel very good when it happened, but it would be over quickly and that afterward, she could have a lollipop and wear some lipstick (her favorite treat). I told her she could cry if she wanted but she would have to stay very still if she wanted the lipstick. Brooke sat on my lap hugging me with my arms over hers keeping her still and leaving her back exposed as the test site. She cried but stayed very still and when it was over, quickly hopped off my lap requesting her reward. I gave her the lollipop and applied the bright red lipstick to her tiny lips. She smacked her lips together with delight before racing to her daddy in the waiting room.

The results of the tests showed what we'd feared, that Brooke tested positive to almost everything in her environment and diet. A list of food families and environmental controls was handed to me. Dust, pollens, horses, cats, birds, wheat, most grains, eggs, nuts, legumes, chicken, beef, oranges, peaches, milk—the allergens seemed endless. As I read the list at home, I began to cry. The list was so long and overwhelming.

Brooke's dainty nursery would have to be stripped and her diet would have very little variety. Wanting to be the best mom possible, I began to attack the list with fervor, but I soon started to feel that, despite my best efforts, I would never measure up.

By this time our lives had become consumed by this little person. Her allergies were so numerous it was hard to find something to feed her. Countless nights Brooke coughed and gagged as I rocked her in the lonely darkness of her room. My tiny princess grew up in doctors' office waiting rooms, emergency rooms and hospitals. She was taking numerous daily medications and as a result experienced long periods of chemically induced hyperactivity. Yet she toddled through life quite unaware that it should be any different.

Asthma complicated everything, even the usual problems of life. While pregnant with our fourth child, I was restricted to bed rest. Somehow I was supposed to juggle the bed rest prescribed to ensure the good health of a child as yet unborn, with the needs of two healthy, active boys and a daughter whose asthma demanded medical intervention almost daily. She wheezed and coughed so much, I began to accept it as normal breathing for Brooke. I was very tired, and though my husband hired a high school girl to come in and clean once a week, I felt like I was stuck somewhere in the twilight zone. I needed relief.

So I prayed. It was my friends at church who picked up the pieces of my life and took care of washing my laundry, cooking meals and sustaining me in a time of need. When we sold our home to move closer to Dale's work and the doctor's office, our church members packed, cleaned, then moved and helped unpack and feed our family.

Brooke was hospitalized repeatedly for asthma. We worked closely with her doctor to find medications which would not upset her sensitive stomach. We noticed other drug side effects as well, such as crying jags, drastic behavior changes, headaches and stomach pain. Trying to break the cycle of her illness was like trying to tunnel through a mountain with an ice pick. Though I did not understand any logical reason behind the madness of my life, I was sure God knew and I began to trust that in time, I too would understand.

In the meantime, I had work to do. I gave birth to Brooke's little brother just after she turned two. We were renting a house while our new home was being built so time I would have spent feathering the nest was spent reading everything about asthma I could get my hands on.

The bookstores and library offered little help. It was already apparent to me that the books on the shelves were grossly outdated, and I found no written material on the practical aspects of raising a child with asthma. What I knew about asthma, I learned by asking my doctor questions and reading medical journals she kept on her shelf at the office.

I didn't know anyone else who had a child with asthma. When I asked Brooke's doctor if there was anyone else like us out there, she said she didn't have any other patients as seriously ill as Brooke. Efforts to contact a support group proved fruitless as none existed in our area. So I tucked my troubles inside, determined that, with the help of my doctor, we would exhaust all the alternatives.

One particular day, when Brooke was almost five years old, she came into my room crying. When I asked her the reason for her tears, she replied, "I don't know, I just can't stop crying and I really don't know why."

I suspected the source of her tears was her medication because wide mood swings can follow the introduction of specific medications.

I rocked Brooke until she fell asleep. I was beginning to hate the medicines my daughter required. They made her heart "bleep" as she called it. They made her stomach and head hurt and now they made her cry. When she awoke she felt better but after her next dose of meds the tears and complaints started again. All this pain, and she was still wheezing.

She became pale and dark circles ringed her eyes. "Mommy, I am tired and I can't stop crying again." I sat on the edge of the bed and cried my quiet, sad tears, too. Had everything been in vain all these years? Were there answers to this problem we could live with? There had to be someone out there doing something new for people with asthma and allergies. I was sure of it but did not know how to find that help.

I blew my nose and reached for the phone. I called our doctor. She was not in the office at the time so I spoke to the nurse practitioner. "I know it is the medication. Is there something I can give her to counteract the constant tears and stomach pain?" The nurse spoke with the doctor on call while I waited, hoping for an answer that could be found in a pill. Brooke was wheezing and still sobbing as she lay on my lap. "Mrs. Sander, I'm sorry but the doctor said there is nothing you can give her to counteract the depression or the pain, but let me suggest that you continue to hold her and talk her through it. In a couple of hours she should be her normal self again."

It was not the answer I wanted to hear. I thought, "How in

the world does she expect me to hold this weeping, wheezing child for the next few hours with three other children running around and a husband at work?" I called Dale but the most he could offer was encouragement.

Brooke didn't get better physically although the symptoms of depression did wear off by the end of the day. By the next day, Saturday, it was evident that Brooke was in serious trouble with her asthma. She was weak, pale and curled up in a little ball. Her little chest heaved and when her eyes met mine, my heart was pierced. Dr. McGee met me in the emergency room.

Despite her best efforts, Dr. McGee could not break the attack in the emergency room using breathing treatments and adrenaline injections. She needed an intravenous form of theophylline called aminophylline.

Dr. McGee assured me she would stay with Brooke and would stop the aminophylline if she saw a bad reaction. The IV drip was started and within two hours Brooke was again curled up in the fetal position crying quiet, sorrowful tears and growing sicker by the moment. The aminophylline was stopped and replaced with steroids and Brooke was admitted to the hospital again.

Upon Brooke's discharge from the hospital, a follow-up visit with the doctor was scheduled. I had read everything I could find about asthma and had come to the conclusion that even though we were seeing very good doctors we needed *something more.* I was prepared to discuss this with Brooke's doctor. While waiting for her in the examination room, I took a recent copy of *Annals of Allergy* off her shelf and noticed that three of the doctors listed inside were in the Washington, D.C., area. When Dr. McGee walked in the door I clasped the journal in my hand and asked her what she thought about my calling these doctors to see if they had any additional information to offer. She agreed and said that she would make some calls as well.

I called all three doctors but could reach only two of them. One, Dr. Michael Kaliner at the National Institutes of Health (NIH) in Bethesda, Maryland, listened to our story and commented that our doctor was doing everything that could be done that he was aware of and that, unfortunately, NIH did not have a pediatric study program at that time. I called Dr. Michael Sly at Children's Hospital in Washington, D.C., and he too said that Brooke's medical regimen sounded good and that no, they did not have anything new to offer children with her severity. I called Dr. Joseph Bellanti's office at Georgetown University Hospital, but he was not in.

A couple of days later Brooke had to go back to see Dr. McGee and I told her about the phone calls. Though I still had hopes of reaching Dr. Bellanti, Dr. McGee had actually gotten through to him. He told her of a drug study program being conducted at the Georgetown University Hospital and referred us to one of his fellows, Dr. Martha Vetter White. She handed me a white slip of paper with the name and phone number written in pencil. "I think Brooke will qualify for the study, but the requirements are pretty strict."

I did not care. I knew that we were running out of options fast and I feared for the life of my child. I found it difficult to imagine Brooke participating in Scouts, going on picnics or enjoying an amusement park. I found it hard to imagine her ever wearing a beautiful white wedding gown or being healthy enough to bear children. I clutched the piece of paper in my hand and left the office both frightened and confident. Frightened that this, my seemingly last option, might not work and confident that I was doing what I had to do.

The petite blond woman who greeted us looked like everybody's best friend. What a treat it was when she introduced herself as Brooke's doctor. She explained the conditions for acceptance in the program, the object of the study and what would happen if Brooke became too sick to remain in the study.

The drug being tested, ketotifen/Zaditen, had received good reports in Europe where it had been used for ten years but to be approved for use in the United States it was necessary to demonstrate its effectiveness and safety in a test here. That meant that some children would receive a placebo, a look-and-taste-alike drug that has no medicinal value, and some children would receive the real drug. It was a "double blind" study, which meant that neither the doctor nor the family would know if a child was on a placebo until after the seven-month trial period was over.

During that time, we would have to use a peak flow meter (described in Chapter 6) to chart her "blows" twice daily. I would have to chart her "daily medical diary," which tracked her health as well as the medications she was taking. The only reported side effect of the medication was drowsiness, which disappeared after adjusting the dose. Some of Brooke's other medications were adjusted and all my questions were answered. It was explained that if Brooke required more than two bursts (dosing periods) of steroids (an anti-inflammatory medication which could mask the study objectives) or more than two hospitalizations during this time she would be removed from the study. After several tests Brooke qualified for the study program and my hope was renewed. Temporarily.

During the seven-month study period that followed, Brooke required two hospitalizations and two bursts of steroids. Keeping her healthy during this period was extremely difficult. I became discouraged because I feared if she was taking the real thing and not the placebo, we were fresh out of options.

Brooke began taking the "open label medication" or the real thing immediately after the seven months ended. I was not to receive confirmation on whether or not she was one of the "placebo kids" for six more weeks. Imagine my delight as I noticed subtle improvements such as skin clearing, less wheezing, fewer viral and bacterial infections, less vulnerability to allergens and, most impressive, improved and stabilized peak flow meter readings. Her chart showed her asthma was becoming stabilized and so were all other allergy symptoms. Her chart proved to me that she'd been on the placebo and that now she was on "the real thing."

We began to understand her asthma better and were even able to prevent many attacks. We learned to identify triggers and early warning signals and how and when to respond to them. With the wheezing under control, we were able to distinguish other physical problems, some of which contributed to her asthma. For example, we began to understand the impact of chronic sinus infections on her asthma. After visiting yet another specialist, an otolaryngologist (better known as an ENT or OTO doctor), a plumbing problem with her sinuses was diagnosed and a treatment plan was established to try to control the infections until she was old enough to have them operated on. One unexpected result of clearing her impacted sinuses was that Brooke's hearing improved tremendously.

It was only last year that we began to understand the reasons for her stomach pain and sensitivities. She was recently referred to a gastroenterologist at Georgetown University Hospital in Washington, D.C., and diagnosed as having three ulcers and gastritis. The cause is not known entirely, but a combination of factors, including food allergies, family history, the stress of multiple physical problems and possibly medications set the stage for the condition. In my humble opinion, I think asthma is easier to manage than ulcers. However, that may simply be because this condition is still new to me.

During those first six years of Brooke's life, medical technology and pharmacology took some great leaps forward. Inhaled steroids were developed and albuterol (a bronchodilator option with fewer side effects and a longer period of action than other bronchodilators at that time) became FDA approved. Diagnostic tests became more sophisticated. Though it did not apply to Brooke because she could not tolerate theophylline in any dosages, theophylline became available in a variety of time-released formulas and dose sizes.

For the first time Brooke's asthma was not controlling our lives and it was because good doctors were prescribing good medications and teaching me how to respond properly to early warning signals and triggers and to take environmental precautions in our home. I knew that if control was possible for Brooke, it was possible for the majority of children who suffer with asthma today.

I wanted to share the good news of asthma management and for the first time since Brooke was born, I felt I was able to reach out to others. As a writer and busy mother, I felt I could best reach out to others through the written word. I believed that a newsletter would be the most effective, inexpensive means of communication. The hurdle that lay before me was obtaining Dale's support for the project.

We'd mini-vacationed at Dale's brother's beach place for a long weekend and were on the way home again. Mike and Dan, my oldest boys, were in the back of the van. Brooke and Joe occupied the middle bench seat. The kids were wrapped up in their own conversations. I shed my shoes, propped my bare feet on the dash, took a deep breath and started to tell Dale about what I'd been thinking.

"We've learned a lot about Brooke's asthma," I said.

"M-m-m." Dale nodded.

I told him that I wanted to write a newsletter for parents of children who have asthma. It would start as a local endeavor, I explained. Then after a few years, it would expand to a national newsletter. I'd figured it would cost me very little as long as I typed it myself and used rub-on headings. I'd arranged to borrow the copier at a friend's store in town and figured my major cost would be postage. Charging eight dollars a year for twelve issues, I expected to make enough money to cover expenses and pay for Brooke's and Joey's school bill. This would allow me to quit my part-time job and write the newsletter out of my home.

As Dale listened to my idea, he played devil's advocate. A few miles later, he gave his blessing and support on one condition, that my little idea did not break the family budget.

I sat down at my dilapidated Smith Corona. I rolled in the first piece of paper and the words started to pour out. I placed my rub-on lettering over each column between preparing kids' snacks and folding loads of laundry. I asked Dr. White to edit the newsletter for medical accuracy. *MA Report*, the sole publication and purpose of Mothers of Asthmatics, Inc., was born.

I mailed sample copies of the November issue to about seventy-five doctors' offices in the Washington, D.C., area. One of Brooke's doctors had invited me to a medical conference in Washington at which the experimental drug Brooke was taking would be discussed. I ran off a few extra copies of *MA Report* and put them in my briefcase.

At the conference, I met Mr. Johns, an official from Sandoz, the pharmaceutical company that manufactures the experimental drug that Brooke was taking. I introduced myself to him just before the meeting started and handed him a copy of the newsletter. I tried to listen to the doctors making the presentations, but I could see over Mr. Johns's shoulder that he was reading the newsletter. Suddenly I wondered how I would respond if he simply smiled and said, "What a nice newsletter. Keep up the good work," indicating he obviously thought it was a homespun production.

My watch indicated I had only fifteen minutes left before I had to get home for my children. As I was in the middle of these anxious thoughts, he (or the manager) turned and whispered, "This newsletter is great. Can we talk?" He pointed to the exit doors and I nodded.

Once outside, Mr. Johns began asking questions about my marketing plans and projected expenses. I answered his questions as best as I could. Then he suggested I fly to New Jersey in a few weeks to discuss how Sandoz could help Mothers of Asthmatics. I smiled so hard I thought my face was going to break. He walked back into the meeting and I got lost in the hotel trying to find the parking lot.

It turned out that Sandoz did indeed provide start-up funds for the newsletter, no strings attached. How was I going to spend the money? I needed a lawyer, a desk, some paper and paper clips to start with.

A reporter from the Fairfax *Journal* came out to the house to report on the newsletter and took some pictures. This was our first media encounter and from that one article alone, distribution of the newsletter grew to nine states.

Just about the time my system of tracking subscribers was overwhelming me, a letter from Debbie Scherrer arrived in the mail. "I am a 'retired' bank manager mother of two children with asthma. I have the time and ability to manage your mailing list on my home computer and would like to help." I called her right away to set up the mailing system.

Others called to volunteer their services and dedication. Equally impressive were their children. They were so excited about their moms being involved in a project that would help them understand asthma better, they often stamped and folded newsletters. Many times they would swap suggestions with each other on how to swallow pills or how to take yucky-tasting medicines. If one child hesitated to use his inhaler before going out to play, the others chided him into compliance.

Other pharmaceutical companies and corporations soon became interested in supporting the newsletter, providing graphics, typesetting and printing, equipment and travel grants so that I could speak to various support groups and get publicity for Mothers of Asthmatics. One pharmaceutical company provided an educational grant for *Asthma and Allergies in the School: The Importance of Cooperative Care*, a patient/educator education video accompanied by two special editions of *MA Report*. MA, Inc., grew. (See Resources section at the back of this book.)

Our message was clear. Asthma, mild, moderate or severe, can be managed. We must become aware of early warning signals, triggers and what to do at the first sign of trouble. We must prepare, think ahead, adapt and adjust. We must work with doctors who know how to manage asthma using current methods of treatment. We must teach our children and weave coping skills into their daily lives.

Asthma doesn't have to cripple or kill our children. Asthma, like any other adversity, can draw families closer together, create an opportunity to understand the suffering of others and give a greater appreciation of life.

I founded Mothers of Asthmatics in the belief that for the first time in history medical technology presents us with options we can live with. I have seen with my own eyes the beauty and freedom of controlled asthma free from the side effects and limitations of management techniques of the past.

Today, Brooke is managing her asthma on a daily basis. Her treatment plan is preventive with early intervention as required. Treatment therapies of yesteryear took the "let's wait and see if the attack progresses" approach. Thankfully, this is not the best that medical technology has to offer today. But more on that later.

Brooke is bright (even if it is her mom saying it, it is still true). She plays the piano, loves to swim and plays basketball with the county league. Her teachers describe her as assertive and tenacious but always sensitive to the needs of others. She is a normal kid though and gets in the usual number of sibling feuds with her brothers.

These days Brooke finds her few stomach ulcers of far greater concern than preventing the asthma attacks. In fact, Brooke's attitude about asthma under control is "having asthma's really not so bad, once you get the hang of it."

There are far worse diseases and adversities in life than asthma. Yes, we have adjustments to make and some of those can be very difficult, but we have everything to gain by trying.

Asthma under control is worth the effort. It really is.

CHAPTER 2

ASTHMA BASICS

WHEN I GOT MY FIRST CAR, MY FATHER showed me how to use jumper cables, check the oil and pump gasoline. This newly gained knowledge did not make me a mechanic but it did provide a basic foundation to build on as necessary.

If this is your first experience with asthma, you will need some foundation information, too. This foundation will include some basics about asthma physiology, how to separate fact from fiction, medications and how to recognize a good doctor when you see one. This is a foundation that you will build upon each day as you work toward the goal of controlled asthma.

The first step to mastering asthma is to understand it better. This chapter will provide some of the basic facts about asthma, but remember, this is a book about parenting children with asthma. If you want detailed information about the physiology and medical management of asthma, read *Asthma: The Complete Guide to Self-Management of Asthma and Allergies for Patients and Their Families,* by Allan M. Weinstein, M.D.

Before you read any further, *parents who don't have asthma or heart disease* should try this simulated asthma attack. Run in place for two minutes. Then, while pinching your nose, place a straw in your mouth and see how long you can breathe that way. Does it cause you to feel anxious? Panicky? It ought to.

Fortunately, you can remove the straw and normal breathing will be restored. Relief from asthma is not that easy. It requires a cooperative effort between patient and doctor to develop a comprehensive plan for asthma management. However, *controlled asthma is possible.*

Asthma affects the **airways,** the tubes through which the air you breathe travels to the **air sacs** where your blood is oxygenated. (In contrast, emphysema is a destructive disease of the air sacs.) Surrounding the airways are smooth muscles that constrict or spasm during an asthma attack, squeezing the airway from the outside. They are involuntary muscles, which means that we cannot consciously make them contract and expand the way we can flex our biceps and other voluntary muscles. (Though there are certainly differences, any woman who has ever experienced labor knows the power of involuntary smooth muscles!) This tightening, called bronchoconstriction, makes it more difficult for air to flow through the lungs.

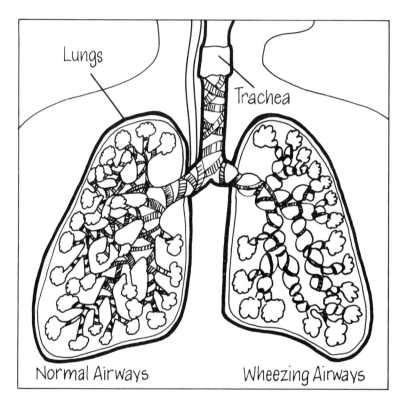

Look at the illustration of the airways. During an asthma attack (or episode or flare as it is sometimes called), fluid leaks from blood vessels, filling the cells that make up the lining of the airways and causes swelling. If the attack is prolonged, inflammatory cells from the bloodstream also leak out with the fluid. Now we have an air tube which is being squeezed from the outside and is puffing up inside, leaving even less room for the air to pass through. The wheeze that characterizes asthma is the high-pitched whistling sound the air makes as it tries to force its way through the narrowed opening.

The airways are lined with cilia (tiny hairlike projections whose function is to move mucus along) and a thin layer of mucus. The mucus lubricates the air we breathe and traps tiny foreign particles we inevitably breathe in, and the cilia promptly escort them out of our system (we either cough them out or swallow them). In an asthma flare, however, far too much mucus is produced, and it gets thick and gooey. So not only does the air have to pass through a narrowed tube, but it must also make its way through a sticky mess. Sometimes mucus globs together forming mucus plugs that block portions of the airway, trapping stale air in the little air sacs where the air is supposed to perform its task of delivering oxygen to the blood and removing the waste product, carbon dioxide.

Degrees of bronchoconstriction vary from mild to moderate to severe. Its occurrence ranges from infrequent (once annually) to frequent (once a month) to chronic (several times or more a month). The combination of degree and frequency of bronchoconstriction determines asthma's impact on your child's life.

Perhaps your child has a mild episode of asthma once or twice a year. During each bout, persistent, nonproductive coughing responds to a bronchodilating-type medication. The entire episode lasts three or four days and there is no further problem. This type of asthma is less likely to have a great impact on the family than a mild coughing asthma that occurs nightly for weeks or months (which is chronic, mild asthma). However, the daily activities of the child who has chronic severe asthma (and of the child's family) will be drastically curtailed unless asthma is controlled.

To control asthma is to reduce its impact on the lives it touches. Control comes through a variety of means but most often by removing precipitators (triggers) of asthma attacks, responding appropriately to early warning signals (EWS), understanding how to administer appropriate medications and how soon they should take effect, and communicating effectively with a doctor qualified and experienced in treating asthma. Sometimes gaining control over asthma is as simple as removing an offending food from the diet or a pet from the home. However, controlling asthma is usually more complex.

Asthma can be associated with allergies, but can also be present without them. Asthma is sometimes accompanied by eczema (usually characterized by inflamed, itchy skin) and nasal polyps (fluid-filled bulbous sacs in the nasal airways). Sinus infections, colds and other viral infections, often precede asthma attacks. Many people have asthma only when they exercise.

Regardless, the most difficult time for many parents of children with asthma is between diagnosis and control. During this period, which can last days, weeks, months or years, parents have to adapt to a new world and learn a new vocabulary of asthma and allergy terms like "triggers" and "early warning signals," "allergens," "self-management" and "control." As parents learn how to apply this information to their own children, they will be taking the first steps toward getting asthma under control.

And once asthma is controlled, management becomes fairly routine.

TRIGGERS

Asthma is usually genetically engineered at the time of conception. Unless a person is genetically predisposed to asthma, exposure to any of the triggers in the list that follows will not induce an attack. However, to the person who suffers with asthma, a close encounter with a trigger can activate breathing problems. In some cases, exposure to a trigger can be life-threatening.

Many things can trigger or initiate an asthma attack. But remember, triggers do not *cause* asthma. Triggers, which can be allergic or nonallergic, activate a chain reaction of events that lead to the asthma attack. Depending on the trigger and sensitivity of the individual, a reaction (asthma attack, hives, etc.) can occur immediately after exposure to a trigger or be delayed.

Children with asthma may react to one or more of the following triggers but you should not assume that everything listed will trigger your child's asthma:

THE MOST COMMON TRIGGERS

Colds and Infections
Exercise
Allergy
    Molds
    Tree pollen
    Grass pollen
    Certain foods and additives

Animals (dogs, cats, horses and birds are most common)

Climatic Elements
Wind
Rain
Cold air
Other dramatic fluctuations in weather

Medications
Aspirin
"Beta-blockers" (such as those used for heart problems or an eye drop for glaucoma)

Emotions
Laughing
Crying
Holding breath
Hyperventilating

Irritants
Aerosol sprays
Odor
Smoke
Dust
Air pollution
Paint fumes
Perfume

Make a list of your child's triggers and early warning signals. Keep the list in a safe place. If you don't mind marking up your copy of this book, I don't mind either. Simply place a check mark next to each trigger or early warning signal (EWS) that applies to your child. You might want to mark today's date next to each as well. Triggers may change later.

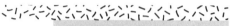

ASTHMA AND ASPIRIN

Approximately 10 percent of people who have asthma are sensitive to aspirin. In these patients, ingestion of aspirin can cause severe asthma attacks that are difficult to control. Therefore most asthma specialists recommend that asthmatics avoid aspirin and medications containing aspirin. **Acetaminophen** (Tylenol, Datril, etc.) should be substituted instead.—Martha V. White, M.D.

EARLY WARNING SIGNALS (EWS)

Early warning signals differ from triggers in that they tell when an attack or episode of asthma is coming. Sometimes an EWS is as subtle as frequent yawning or as seemingly unrelated as itching on the neck or back. The following list contains all the EWS I know about, but that doesn't mean there couldn't be still others that your child may show. Early warning signals can provide clues for early intervention, so recogniz-

ACCORDING TO PLAN

Asthma management plans don't merely consist of understanding triggers and early warning signals, though these are a vital part. Tests, medications, dietary considerations, environmental changes, communication skills and family coping styles all contribute to the success of an asthma management plan.

Parents and doctors become supersleuths as they learn to anticipate, premedicate and respond to the physical and emotional needs of the child with asthma. Your doctor may have to adjust the asthma management plan several times before it is perfected, so it will be important for you to be able to communicate effectively and accurately. It is worth the effort, as these stories demonstrate:

My son, Kyle, age two, is doing very well. Last winter,

1986–87, was terrible. He was in the hospital in October and remained on medication through July. But the last six months have been a breeze. His asthma attacks were brought on by viruses and since I have learned to recognize the early warning signals and start medications right away, we've only been to the doctor twice this winter. This we can live with! No problem!

Miranda has had asthma for four years. Last year she was in ICU for a week and that week our eleven-year-old dog died. Miranda hasn't had asthma since. All along, it was our dog. The dog always did give her a rash but we had no idea it was giving her asthma.

Adam's asthma is triggered by infection. His problems started at two weeks of age and he was hospitalized when three months old due to a serious asthma attack. He did not tolerate theophylline well at that age because he was so small but now he does well on

ing them is a very important part of controlling asthma.

Feels "funny" in the chest
Gets a headache
Eyes look glassy
Irritable
Itchy throat
Cough, especially at night
Sneezy
Runny nose
Pale
Tired
Wants to be alone
Mopey
Dark circles under eyes
Head stopped up
Restless
Nightmares
Waking up at night
Night cough
Reduced peak flow meter readings (more on peak flow meters later).

GASTROESOPH-AGEAL REFLUX

Gastroesophageal reflux is another physical condition which can trigger attacks, especially at night. Put simply, acid from the stomach leaks back up, irritating the lining of the esophagus, since it is not equipped to handle acid as the stomach does. Occasionally some of this material is inhaled into the airways. Either circumstance can trigger a reaction that starts the attack.

Most children respond favorably to antacids and elevating the head of the bed to get gravity to keep the stomach acid where it belongs, while some children must have surgery to remedy the problem. Read *Asthma: The Complete Guide* by Dr. Allan M. Weinstein for more information.

A STICKY SITUATION

In many children with asthma, postnasal drip from rhinitis (rhin—nose; itis—inflammation) or sinusitis (sinus inflammation) may be irritating the airways and triggering asthma flares. Doctors used to prescribe antiasthma medications but did not prescribe antihistamines at the same time. However, new research has shown most antihistamines do not interfere with asthma medications and can help to counteract some of the allergic triggers. Elevating the bed and using a humidifier if the air is

theophylline, Intal (with a nebulizer) and Alupent. Adam is now fifteen months old and we seem to have things under control. Eczema was a real problem, too, but we're even learning how to handle that, too.

Kyle, Miranda and Adam have asthma, which affected their lives to varying degrees before their parents were able to gain control. Kyle's mom learned how to respond to an early warning signal, which allowed her to prevent the asthma attacks from occurring. Miranda's mom discovered the source of her daughter's asthma when the allergen, in this case, the family dog, died, and now Miranda no longer requires daily medications. Adam's mom learned to cope with a new routine which involved medications and understanding triggers, too.

The important thing parents must remember is that well-controlled asthma doesn't happen by accident. It takes an active decision on the part of the parents to obtain the best asthma care possible for their

dry (as in the wintertime) also may help to stop the drip.

child. It takes a willingness to follow the plan according to the doctor's instructions. Effective asthma management plans require making changes and adjusting. However, once asthma is controlled, keeping it that way is rather routine.

MANY FACES OF ASTHMA

As I mentioned before, asthma is often as individual as a fingerprint. There are varying degrees of frequency and severity. Usually the child with moderate or severe asthma is easily identified as having a problem when, ironically, the child with mild asthma is often overlooked. These kids and their parents are the Rodney Dangerfields of asthma. Most often, they just "don't get no respect."

The following story, called "Mild Asthma: Major Problem" by Debbie Scherrer, illustrates this point very well.

My story is very different from most you hear about asthma. Aside from infrequent attacks which resulted in only one trip to the emergency room, the tale of my two children who have asthma is not a dramatic one. It's about two children with relatively mild asthma. The details would put you to sleep. However boring, it's a story of years of confusion, frustration, loss of sleep, multiple visits to doctors, trying desperately to do the best for my children yet feeling there must be something more because somewhere along the way I had lost control to this "ugly thing" called asthma. However, in reality, there are thousands of you who can identify with Greg and Lesley's version of asthma.

For us the "attacks" are few and far between (thank you, God!). Don't get me wrong, but in a very strange way, there's a kind of satisfaction when they occur. As painful as it is to watch my children having trouble, when I say there's a "satisfaction," I mean that at least with a severe attack you get action! Know what I mean? You carry your child into the emergency room and you get immediate attention. Even family and friends sit up and take notice when they see the "real thing" with their own eyes. It is dramatically evident that you need help and there are lots of folks around to help you through it.

The other side of asthma is the one we live with most of the time. It's the boring, wear-you-down-slowly, drive-you-crazy, chronic mild form of asthma. It may be as subtle as a dry, hacking cough that lasts for weeks or months. Or it may be mild flares every night that rob you of sleep and sanity while everyone who sees your child during the day (the doctor, friends and relatives, etc.) sees only a child who is the picture of health. After a while you stop trying to tell these people about your asthma troubles because they're beginning to look at you strangely and whisper words behind your back like "overprotective" and "all in her head." (Or could it be you're becoming a little paranoid from lack of sleep?)

Let's talk about that cough. Those of you who've experienced it know just what I mean! That hacking cough that may not seem too distressing to the doctor who hears it for five minutes while he performs his examina-

tion (which reveals no wheezing at the moment, clear lungs, throat, ears, etc.). He may not understand the desperation that makes my voice quiver when I plead for him to do something about it, unless he is sensitive enough to realize that I've lived with that "harmless little cough" day and night till I'm ready to scream.

I once timed Greg's cough. He couldn't go ten seconds without a little cough. That's six times a minute, 360 times an hour . . . it's too depressing to carry it any further. After a while, the sound of each cough physically makes my stomach hurt. Each cough pounds the message "you need to do more" into my sleep-starved zombie brain. Yet the doctor is unimpressed. Instead of concern and support, I faced an attitude of "just be glad that's all you've got to deal with."

Yes, mild asthma can be a major problem. The urgency that galvanizes everyone into determined action to combat an acute attack is often replaced by ambivalence in the case of chronic mild asthma. Parents and even some doctors often misunderstand the problem and a lack of treatment results. This course of inaction sometimes works out okay, as the mild asthma goes away on its own. The danger lies in the fact that many times a case of mild asthma is merely a warning sign that if left untreated will develop into an acute attack. The frustrations of mild asthma out of control are very real. It's both physically and emotionally exhausting.

For years I put up with the situation, grateful at least that the frightening attacks were controlled, and thinking that this was as much as I could hope for. Finally (with a lot of help from MA), I realized that I was selling myself and my kids short. Asthma (even mild asthma) can be controlled! You don't have to put up with the *mild wheezes, the dry cough, or the nighttime flares. There are answers for all these problems, and a good doctor will help you find them. Just because the problem is not life-threatening is no reason to settle for less than top-notch health care.*

I'm pleased to say that our story has a happy ending. We made a change to a wonderful doctor whose insight and compassion have made a world of difference. With her guidance and aggressive treatment, the coughs and the nightly flares are practically nonexistent, and when they do arise we know what to do. The weeks on end of sleepless nights are nothing more than a bad memory. Take it from me—control is worth the effort. Go for it!

Understanding the physiology and responding properly to triggers and early warning signals is important for all families affected by chronic asthma—whether it is mild, as in the case of Debbie's children, or severe, as in Brooke's situation.

Asthma is a complex problem, and parents can often become discouraged trying to understand it. My best advice to parents is to try to learn and adapt, one day at a time. Keeping a daily health diary can help.

KEEPING A DIARY

By keeping a daily diary of your child's symptoms, peak flow meter readings (see Chapter 6) and medications, you and your doctor will begin to see the pattern of events that lead into an asthma flare. Your doctor will then be able to make adjustments to your asthma management plan that respond to symptoms soon enough to halt the attack in its earliest stages. Remember: A good asthma management plan is one that consists of prevention, early intervention and a strategy for responding to crisis.

It may take a while to establish a pattern, especially if asthma symptoms are not currently well controlled. However, once asthma is controlled, you will see a more stabilized daily record. Don't be tempted to slack off with record keeping when your child is having a good spell. If you do, you will not be able to see the attack coming at the earliest opportunity to intervene.

Make copies of the following chart from The Asthma Organizer (see Resources) to track your child's daily symptoms.

Your response to asthma will be directly related to the degree to which it interrupts your life. It is also true that many parents wear blinders of adjustment to compromised living, thereby denying their child achievement of his or her personal goals with parental encouragement. It is one thing to hurt for our children who have asthma and another thing to help them overcome it.

We are the voice of our children in the adult world. As they grow, we need to teach them to respect and control their asthma. It is only through knowledge that we overcome fear. We must teach our children the things that we learn and then trust them to put the information to good use when they are grown.

Be ready to learn. Read. Talk to your doctor and nurse. Talk to teachers and school nurses.

Yes, there is a life beyond asthma, and by concentrating your efforts on getting asthma under control *right now,* you are headed toward that life where you can say, as one mother recently did, "Though Davey still has asthma, the fear and heartache are behind us like a bad dream."

HOME DIARY #_____

Name _____

Date from ____ to ____ Next Scheduled Appointment ____

Rate the categories below using the numbered key as follows:

Excellent 0, Very Good 1, Good 2, Fair 3, and Poor 4.

DATE															
Activity Level															
Coughing															
Wheezing															
Sleep															
Nose															
Overall Health Assessment															
PEAK FLOW READINGS															
A.M.															
P.M.															
Miscellaneous (Use for weather, AQI, etc.)															
MEDICATIONS															
1. _____															
2. _____															
3. _____															
4. _____															
5. _____															
6. _____															

Use this space to record any questions, suspected early warning signals, possible triggers or anything you wish to discuss with your doctor.

_____

_____

_____

_____

_____

Please record the dates of any *unscheduled* office visits, after-hours treatments, emergency room visits and/or hospitalizations occurring within the dates of this diary page. Please record your impression of the events which led up to the unscheduled visit. (Events can include triggers, activities, etc.)

Date   **Events**

_____   _____

             _____

_____   _____

             _____

_____   _____

             _____

_____   _____

             _____

What did you learn from this unscheduled visit that may help you to prevent the next one?

_____

_____

_____

_____

_____

CHAPTER 3

MYTHS AND OLD WIVES' TALES

I N YOUR JOURNEY TO ASTHMA UNDER CONTROL, YOU will likely encounter old wives' tales and advice from well-meaning people who don't know what they're talking about. Some myths are long standing, others misrepresent current information. Many asthma myths are still in books, magazines and tabloids today. Beware. Be wise.

Some of these myths and old wives' tales follow, but you may have heard a few that I have not:

- Asthma is the result of a psychological disorder. It's all in your head.
- Asthma is the result of a poor mother and child relationship.
- Children grow out of asthma.
- Move to Arizona.
- Pet a Chihuahua.
- Asthma doesn't kill anyone anymore.
- Asthma doesn't require medical treatment.
- Asthma isn't serious anymore.

MYTH #1: IT'S ALL IN YOUR HEAD

My father collects old books. Every once in a while, he comes across a medical book or magazine with asthma information. One such book he gave me, *The Complete Common Sense Medical Adviser,* by V. Pierce, M.D., published in 1918, helped me to understand more about the first myth on our list, that asthma is the result of a psychological problem. This is not the first record of this belief, it just happens to illustrate the perception and definition of asthma at that time:

> *As to the exact pathological condition in this malady, opinions differ. Some physicians consider it a disease of the nervous system, others, of the blood, others, of the bronchial tubes, while not a few believe it to be dependent upon some disease of the stomach, heart, liver, kidneys, or due to urinary affections, or "female weakness." Respecting all these diseases of special organs, it is evident that any complication and particularly one*

that is debilitating or causes irritation of the nervous system will increase its severity. This important fact we keep constantly in view in our treatment, and prescribe remedies to remove all complications.

A sudden fright, unfavorable news, grief, loss of property, etc., circumstances which affect the mind and nervous system, almost invariably throw the phthisical [asthmatic] *into a paroxysm. Nervines* [barbituates, narcotics, addictive compounds] *are demanded, particularly if the case be a chronic one and we see that they are carefully and properly prepared and supplied, and in such a form as to be exactly fitted to the temperament and constitution.*

The doctors did the best they could with the information they had. Because they were unable to observe the physiology and chemistry of the immune system that produce an attack, they assumed that the symptoms and triggers of asthma were in truth the causes. If the patient was anxious about his condition, a sedative was thought to remedy the problem. Those that did not respond to this treatment were thought to have psychological problems, not asthma. Thus the myth.

PSYCHOSOMATIC?

Many well-meaning people blamed my husband for my children's problems (he had asthma first), blamed our house, dog (we gave away our beautiful golden retriever), blamed stress and always said,

Perusing consumer medical guides and asthma books sold in stores today, I found some of these same asthma myths 1980s style. In a recent book on asthma, the author traces the cause of his asthma to a troubled childhood. "At the age of nineteen, I encouraged a reconciliation between my parents, and the family began to communicate again. I often wonder whether I would have developed asthma at all if they had found a way to stay together and battle out their differences in a more constructive way." (He also credits his "cure" of asthma to breathing exercises—we'll talk about these later—but as of today, there are no cures for asthma, including breathing exercises.)

The great danger I see in the large amount of inaccurate reporting or writing today is that people like you and me think that everything we read in print is gospel. So when we read conflicting information, we become confused. Seek out quality information, ask questions and don't settle for nebulous answers. The more you learn about asthma the less susceptible you will be to its myths.

"But your children look so normal." Our entire family has asthma!—Mother in Medina, New York

Asthma and allergies are not psychosomatic. They are real diseases but like many other diseases, they can be worsened by psychic stress. When someone is under psychic stress, there are lots of biochemical changes in the body. The cells that are involved in allergy are influenced by these same biochemical stresses, so that the cells may be more reactive. The other thing that happens is you stimulate the release of chemicals that actually trigger the allergic reaction. Asthma and allergies are not psychological in that the child has the disease and the parent is not responsible for bringing it on, it's that the biochemical environment induced by the psychic stress can make the allergies much worse.—Michael Kaliner, M.D., Section Head, Allergic Disease Section, National Institutes of Health, Bethesda, Maryland

MYTH #2: ASTHMA IS THE RESULT OF A POOR MOTHER AND CHILD RELATIONSHIP

This theory is still commonly believed in many countries. For example, we received this letter from a mother in Japan:

> *I was so worried about this asthma. My son is now fifteen. The greatest difficulties were that I had to move so very often because of the nature of my husband's job. I could not, therefore, ask a certain doctor to take care of him for an appropriately long period. I had to move from one doctor to another. In Japan, the doctors are more or less considered to be divine. They are to be respected. Many patients are afraid to ask questions or give any kind of opinion. His attitude is "You don't need to know or understand. All you have to do is obey me."*
>
> *There are many good and bad points in the way the Japanese doctors are. However, I really wanted to know the reason for his care and treatment or medications and all the injections. Most Japanese doctors do not like "smart" women.*
>
> *Moreover, many think that asthma is caused by the overattention or lack of attention (either) on the part of the mothers. A few years ago, a book called* A Mother-Originated Disease: Asthma *became one of the best sellers. Those are the reasons why I began to study asthma myself. I even got a doctor's degree in health science last year at Tokyo University. My son, in spite of his asthma,*

became a rugby player and was even in the newspaper several times because his team at high school was chosen as a representative team for the prefecture.

The mother and child association as a cause of asthma was explored during the fifties and sixties by psychiatrists. The efforts were joined by other physicians. The results were that mothers were pegged, categorized and sorted into types. Nowhere in any of the literature was any importance placed on the father's relationship with the child. However, the mother theory was so popular that dozens of medical papers were published describing the "asthmatogenic" mother. She was passive, aggressive, compliant, argumentive, domineering, controlling and overprotective. Try as they might, the doctors could not differentiate the asthmatogenic mother from any other mother of a child with a chronic illness, nor were they ever able to document a laboratory-controlled mother-induced asthma attack.

Some of the reports categorized parenting abilities and personalities and tried to compare them with those of mothers of children without asthma. Some tried to find a cause and effect relationship between parenting abilities and the severity of children's asthma. After eight years of unsubstantiated and inconclusive findings, the subject lost the interest of investigators but the damage had only begun.

Chronic illness brings out the best and worst in everyone. As parents, we sacrifice sleep at night and spend our days in doctors' offices and emergency rooms. To suppose for one moment that we enjoy it makes me see red. Anyway, it just so happens that this was another myth, this one perpetuated by medical science.

MYTH #3: CHILDREN GROW OUT OF ASTHMA

Some myths, like this one, are meant to reassure parents. Many fine doctors today continue to tell parents that "children grow out of asthma" when what they really mean is that asthma can go into remission as children grow older. Asthma is not like a pair of shoes. "Kids with asthma don't grow out of it any more than they grow out of the color of their eyes," according to Bob Lanier, M.D., a pediatric allergist in Fort Worth, Texas.

A CHILD'S VIEW

I think the worst thing was waiting to grow out of asthma when I was twelve like the doctor said I would. When I didn't I was so disappointed, like I'd failed or something.—Fourteen-year-old girl, Rockville, Maryland

One out of every five children has asthma before the age of sixteen. About half of those children with asthma have no symptoms by the time they are fifteen years old. However, there are no guarantees that symptoms in remission won't return at any age. Allergy symptoms that linger, if allowed to progress uncontrolled, can actually reactivate the asthma cycle. Uncontrolled asthma and allergies can lead to poor self-esteem, needless frustration and problems with the psychosocial development of your child. It would be unwise and possibly dangerous to assume that asthma is best managed by waiting for the child to "grow out of it."

Doctors aren't able to predict which particular children will experience a reduction in asthma symptoms and which will not. However, asthma is more likely to persist beyond childhood if: asthma begins when child is under two years of age; allergy is a contributing factor; nasal polyps are present; the child is a boy; and the child has frequent asthma attacks or routine wheezing that is difficult to manage. Asthma that is triggered by virus or infection will many times subside as the child's immune system matures.

WE WERE WRONG

I have a three-year-old girl who gets minor attacks of asthma triggered by colds. She is taking medication daily and has required adrenaline injections at the doctor's office to bring it under control in the past. We thought she had grown out of it this year since it had been about six months since her last attack, but I guess we were wrong.—Mother in Bealton, Virginia

Many people confuse controlled asthma with asthma that is in remission. Controlled asthma requires daily intervention to prevent attacks from occurring. Asthma that is in true remission requires no medication or daily intervention, is not triggered by exposure to allergens and could never be described as "living in spite of asthma."

Many times, we adapt our lives so gracefully that our children barely notice all the preventive measures we take to control their asthma. We run the air filters in the furnace, keep their bedrooms clean, change sheets often, watch their diets carefully and give them their medicines. As they get older and are better at listening to their bodies, we adapt again and symptoms seem to subside.

After adolescence, asthma may return. Our children move

out of the protection of home. They are usually living on limited funds and doing the best they can with what they have. Their new home may not have air-conditioning or an air-filtering system. They probably don't change their sheets as often (pollen and dust mites are two good reasons to do this often). They may spend more time around people who smoke or even begin smoking themselves. And if asthma has been in remission long enough, they probably don't respect diet restrictions. The absence of the little things that we do as parents—which our children are either not aware of or don't understand the importance of—can pile up and reactivate the asthma and allergy symptoms.

MYTH #4: MOVE TO ARIZONA

We have quite a number of subscribers from Arizona who can testify that Arizona is not a paradise for asthmatics. On the other hand, some people do experience relief of symptoms with a move to a different climate. Others trade the old allergies for new ones. I've received calls and letters from parents who have moved to another climate and found relief. I have also received calls from people who never had any trouble with asthma or allergies until they moved to their new location.

The best argument for making an asthma-related move is to avoid otherwise unavoidable triggers such as cold air or high humidity and moldiness. There is no skin test to predict allergies to a new location, but my advice for parents is this: Exhaust every alternative for control with a qualified asthma and allergy specialist before uprooting yourselves. And for goodness' sake, if you do decide to move, leave your allergens behind. Don't bring the cat, dog, indoor plants, the farm, etc.

A word of caution to parents who decide to relocate because of asthma: Please don't lay the burden of such a decision on the shoulders of a child who will most likely feel guilty if the asthma does not improve. Devise a plan that includes adventure, a home and secure employment upon arrival. Chronic asthma and relocating are themselves stressful enough. Avoid additional stress by planning ahead. That includes finding a good pediatrician and asthma specialist before you move.

At one point, we wanted to move to Florida because it seems that Brooke is healthiest there. But the risks to Dale's career were far stronger that the assurance that Brooke would benefit from the move so we opted to stay in Virginia. Today, her asthma is well controlled with minimal medical intervention.

MYTH #5: PET A CHIHUAHUA

Dale's mother and father are wonderful in-laws. They are not given to believing in fairy tales, but I'll never forget when they wanted desperately to buy a Chihuahua for Brooke because two of their friends told them that they'd bought one for their grandchildren who had asthma and after the children petted the dog every day, their asthma went away.

This myth probably got its start in Mexico where it was observed that some children with asthma improved at about the same time as the Chihuahua developed it. The truth is that Chihuahuas are born with a predisposition to respiratory problems. (How's that for a piece of interesting trivia?) If a child experiences a remission of asthma at about the same time as the dog develops it, it is merely coincidence. Fortunately, we were able to dissuade Dale's parents from the purchase. However, I love them for trying.

MYTH #6: ASTHMA DOESN'T KILL ANYONE ANYMORE

Asthma is a serious problem. But there is a tendency for books and journals to make light of the incidence of asthma deaths. It gives me little comfort when I read statistics like, "only one in 500,000 people die of asthma each year." The grief of losing a child to asthma is not softened by the knowledge that he or she was one of the minority. Some books state that asthma deaths are rare and that death is most common among low-income blacks and adolescent males. Does that mean that white parents of female children have little to worry about? Or that race, and economic standing might condemn a child to death? Certainly not.

The vast majority of people who die from an asthma attack today are victims of not getting the help they need early enough in the attack. Most attacks can be predicted hours or sometimes even days in advance by understanding and using a simple and inexpensive device such as a peak flow meter (see Chapter 6). This kind of technology was not widely used until recent years, and even today there are many who are only beginning to understand the freedom such a tool can provide.

A report in the *Journal of Allergy and Clinical Immunology* by the Asthma Mortality Task Force of The American Academy of Allergy and Immunology concluded that "it is almost certain that undertreatment rather than overtreatment" is the probable cause of death in the majority of cases today. "Failure of the patient and physician to recognize a deteriorating clinical condition and over-reliance on inhalers (inhaler abuse) creates a potentially fatal scenario."

Asthma is not an either/or type of disease. You don't *either* live with it *or* die because of it. Far greater are the number of people who cope with it or keep it under control than those who die of it.

It is unrealistic to fear death from asthma any more than you would fear death while driving a car. When you drive, you do so defensively. You and your children wear seat belts and you obey traffic signals. When parenting the child with asthma, do so defensively. Follow your doctor's carefully worded instructions, communicate your concerns and beware of early warning signals. Be prepared for the unexpected.

While Brooke was small, her asthma was out of control almost every day of her life. I focused on helping her live because I was very aware that death was a real possibility. How ironic that her most narrow escape from death occurred after asthma had been well controlled for almost two years, and after she'd been in the emergency room for several hours. Though the aftershock of witnessing our doctor restore breathing for Brooke remains a vivid memory, I do not fear that she will die from asthma. We discussed the events that led to the episode and corrected any chance of ever repeating them. Asthma deaths can happen, but *most* of them can be prevented today.

DON'T TAKE ASTHMA FOR GRANTED

I, too, like many other people, never realized the seriousness and impact of asthma on the family and the child with asthma. Our two-year-old daughter had been hospitalized six times between the age of fourteen months and two years. This was bad enough, but worse was the devastating attack she had in September of 1987.

She started the usual way, with a cold, and I started her on her medicines right away, just like the doctor told me to do. Within twenty-four hours of the beginning of her cold, she was in the emergency room. While in the emergency room, her lungs collapsed and she went into respiratory distress. She was immediately placed on a respirator, requiring it for a week. Because the pressure of the respirator was so great, she developed pneumothorax [holes in the lungs] in three different places and had to have chest tubes inserted to remove the air that had escaped into her chest cavity. At this point,

MYTH #7: ASTHMA DOESN'T REQUIRE MEDICAL TREATMENT

Be wary of anyone who promises a *cure* for asthma with or without medicines. Many parents, myself included, despise giving their children medicines. It seems so unnatural to pump the pills, sprays and liquids into their little bodies. So we search for less invasive means of control.

Some of the ingredients people have used to control asthma the "natural way" are: wheat paste applied to the chest; tomato paste rubbed on the chest; inhaling the steam of herbs; drinking one's own urine; eating chicken livers; standing on one's head; inhaling the smoke of narcotic herbs; enemas; and sucking on peppermint candy. Most of these remedies are left over from medical books of the past when bronchodilators and cough suppressants were concocted from herbs.

Parents must weigh the facts carefully. Most children who have asthma will require medication or some type of medical intervention to control persistent or even occasional symptoms. However, asthma can be controlled well enough today to enable most people with asthma to live full, normal lives without medication side effects.

the doctors didn't feel her chances of surviving were very good. They told us at best, if she did survive, her chances of permanent lung damage were almost 100 percent. Remarkably, after ten days she fully recovered and was released without any permanent damage to her lungs. Needless to say, you never really recover from something like this. Fear of this happening again is part of my daily life.

I didn't write this letter to you to scare parents, but only to say, ''Please don't take asthma for granted. Though it usually doesn't, it can kill.—Mother in Voorheesville, New York

MYTH #8: ASTHMA ISN'T SERIOUS ANYMORE

If asthma isn't serious anymore then we must not need oxygen to breathe.

CHAPTER 4

HOW TO FIND
A GOOD DOCTOR

THROUGHOUT THIS BOOK I STRESS THE IMPOR-
tance of a good asthma management plan that is orchestrated
by a good doctor. Asthma management plans vary from one
person and doctor to another because there is no perfect plan
that benefits all patients all of the time. However, there are
hallmarks that set a good doctor apart from the rest.

A good doctor is one who has certified training in a quality institution.

He or she . . .

> . . . continually updates his or her practice to include scientifically proven methods of asthma management techniques, equipment and pharmacology.
>
> . . . is a good medical detective.
>
> . . . is self-motivated and is a good motivator.
>
> . . . is a good listener. If a doctor listens long enough, the patient will provide the clues needed to prescribe proper therapy.
>
> . . . is an educator of parent and patient.
>
> . . . enables parents and patients to make responsible decisions concerning their daily health care needs without creating an artificial dependence on the doctor.
>
> . . . knows how to use the various tools of the trade and how to teach parents and patients to use them.
>
> . . . includes preventive measures and early intervention in the asthma management plan (rather than treating asthma attacks only after they have progressed to the danger zone).
>
> . . . is not threatened by patients who seek greater knowledge of asthma management techniques.
>
> . . . is not offended if you obtain a second opinion.
>
> . . . coordinates referrals to specialists and communicates with the specialists regarding their findings.

Now that you know what a good doctor is, the burning question is how do you find him or her? I've found that good news spreads fast. Ask around your neighborhood to see what names surface. Try to ascertain the reasons people believe their doctors are the best ones for them, and if their situation matches yours.

Call an asthma-related organization, such as those listed in the Resources section of this book, and ask for recommendations. Also, see if your local hospital has a physicians reference service. Though all pediatricians have patients with asthma, not all pediatricians focus on asthma management. Parents in search of a specialist such as a pulmonologist or allergist should request a listing of pediatric pulmonologists or allergists, and so on. Specialists should also be board-certified in their area of expertise. An example of a specialty organization approved by the American Medical Association is the American Board of Allergy and Immunology.

The following list may help you understand the roles of different specialists:

ALLERGIST/IMMUNOLOGIST—An allergist is a medical doctor who has received specialized training in the recognition, evaluation and treatment of clinical allergy and immunology problems including asthma. Your child's primary care physician may refer you to an allergist if your child's symptoms are not responding to current treatment, if the triggers seem to have an allergy component or if the asthma is increasing in intensity.

OTORHINOLARYNGOLOGIST AND HEAD AND NECK SURGEON—This specialty encompasses head and neck medicine, problems and surgery exclusive of the brain, eyes, teeth, neck and spine. The familiar name of this specialty doctor is ear, nose and throat doctor (ENT). (They're now known as OTO.) Your child may be referred to this doctor for evaluation, treatment of surgery for problems associated with rhinitis, sinusitis, hearing or inner ear problems.

PULMONOLOGIST—A pulmonologist specializes in diseases

of the lungs and airways; the practical management of congenital and structural disorders of the lungs and airways, which include bronchopulmonary dysplasia, cystic fibrosis, recurrent pneumonias, and asthma.

GASTROENTEROLOGIST—A doctor who specializes in diseases and disorders of the stomach and intestines. Your child's doctor may suggest a referral to a gastroenterologist if she suspects that asthma is triggered by gastroesophageal reflux or otherwise persistent or undiagnosed stomach pain (gastritis, ulcers).

IMMUNOLOGIST—A doctor who specializes in the diseases and disorders of the immune system. Many doctors who specialize in allergy also specialize in immunology.

ORTHODONTIST—Your allergist, pediatrician or dentist may refer your child to an orthodontist if problems associated with allergies or nasal obstructions are affecting the development of your child's facial or jawbone structure. Frequently, children who have allergies or enlarged adenoids are mouth breathers. In fact, many children seen by an orthodontist before the age of eleven have allergies and are mouth breathers.

After obtaining the names of prospective doctors, parents can ask to speak to the doctor (or, sometimes even better, the doctor's nurse) over the phone. Some telling questions you may want to ask at this time are:

- Is asthma a psychological disease?
- Will my child outgrow asthma?
- Do you conduct asthma education seminars for your patients or do you know of any resources for asthma education?
- Does the doctor encourage parent participation and home monitoring of asthma?

Try to determine the doctor's treatment philosophy. Some doctors have a "let's wait and see if it goes away" attitude while others are concerned with halting an attack in progress and preventing attacks from occurring.

If a doctor answers your questions completely and to your satisfaction, you may want to schedule a consultation or evaluation for your child.

If you are changing doctors, don't expect the new one to work miracles overnight. Changing doctors may take a little adjusting for you, your child and your doctor. Even so, an aggressive, preventive approach should be included in your doctor's asthma management plan and you should understand the objectives of the chosen means of management.

Considering that asthma and allergies account for the largest number of school and workdays lost each year, and the fact that one in every five Americans suffers from an allergic disease, it would seem that there should be plenty of qualified doctors to go around. But this is just not the case. According to Dr. Michael Kaliner, Section Head, Allergic Diseases, National Institutes of Health, Bethesda, Maryland, as quoted in the Foreword to *Asthma* by Allan M. Weinstein, M.D.:

> *Our medical schools tend to focus upon more dangerous and more exotic diseases than allergy, and many of our finest schools do not even have an allergy program or fail to adequately teach the principals and practice of allergy to students and residents . . . Over the past decade, I have consistently observed that despite the outstanding record of [the highly selected medical] students [who rotate through NIH each year] and the repute of their medical schools, they know and understand very little about allergies and asthma. In fact, my lecture [on basic mechanisms of asthma and allergy] is often the*

only teaching on allergy that these students receive during the clinical phase of their training.

Dr. Kaliner suggests that patients and their families cannot always "rely on their family physician to provide accurate or current information regarding allergy or asthma," and that they should turn to the expertise of the allergist.

Kaliner continues:

> *There has been an explosion of information about asthma and allergies over the past twenty years. Only practitioners with a commitment to excellence in asthma and allergy are likely to be knowledgeable about current concepts and their application to these diseases.*

From my ten years' experience with parenting a child with asthma, I would say that the last five years have seen the greatest changes in asthma management strategies and pharmacology. Doctors who don't keep up condemn their patients to mediocrity at best.

KEEP LOOKING!

All doctors are not created equal. You must be selective. Determine the qualities you want in a doctor and don't settle for less. I know of many doctors who possess all the qualities listed in this chapter. It may take driving to the next town to find one but they are out there.

Not too long ago, a woman phoned me from a small town

in Pennsylvania. Her son has severe asthma and at the time she called, he was in ICU at a major hospital ninety miles from her home. The only allergist in her hometown keeps his pet schnauzer at his office and has a chalkboard (two major triggers for many children with asthma) on the wall in his waiting room. At one of many emergency room visits, her son was turning blue and struggling to breathe. It soon became apparent to the mother that this doctor was unable to decide what action to take, so she took her son to the medical center in the major city closest to her home. The child narrowly survived the incident. Now she gladly drives ninety miles each way to get the routine help her son needs.

There would seem to be no reason that this woman should have to drive her child so far for treatment when a board-certified allergist is located in her hometown. However, after verifying this story before telling it here, it is obvious that this family has no other choice than to seek help outside their area.

Our mail also includes letters like this one from a mother in Long Beach, California: "In your April newsletter, you rate the peak flow meters. I asked our pediatric allergist where to purchase one and he said it sounded like a gimmick and to forget it. Any comment? By the way, we adore him as a physician but we're wondering how current his information is."

From Warwick, Rhode Island, another letter: "When I asked my allergist about a peak flow meter, he said that he would not show us how to use one because it was not worth it. Do you feel that this is a good enough reason to look for another doctor?" Parents should avoid judging the quality or abilities of a physician by his use of a particular device or medication. There are several ways to treat and monitor asthma. It is the doctor's total approach to the management plan that sets him apart.

Peak flow monitoring is a method of measuring or gauging the openness of the airways, a subject that we will address in Chapter Six. Certainly, no one would consider a thermometer a gimmick. It gauges the body's temperature. No one would consider a tire gauge worthless. It measures the air pressure inside the tire. Similarly, the peak flow meter provides objective measurements to which we can respond.

Respected medical institutions such as the National Institutes of Health, Bethesda, Maryland; the National Jewish Center for Immunology and Respiratory Medicine, Denver, Colorado; Johns Hopkins Hospital, Baltimore, Maryland; Geisinger Medical Center, Danville, Pennsylvania, and many others actually teach their patients how to use peak flow meters. Peak flow meters are used by practicing physicians as well as medical researchers to establish the response of the airways to various stimuli and medications. Pharmaceutical companies use them to demonstrate scientifically the effectiveness of their medications. These findings are reported in medical journals which describe how the tests were conducted. Physicians are becoming increasingly aware of peak flow meters, largely as the result of industry influence and grass-roots organizations such as Mothers of Asthmatics, Inc.

Then there was this letter:

> *Our son's pediatrician is a very warm, caring doctor who frequently phones the morning after Aaron has had an attack to find out how he's doing. My son, now seven, truly loves this doctor, who has cared for him for over six years. Aaron has cried in his arms and wiped his nose on his white coat. In spite of his abundant compassion, this pediatrician has an intimidating authoritative manner and offers no education about asthma.*

> *All the information I have has been gathered from reading.*
>
> *Neither our pediatrician nor his two associates use peak flow meters or nebulizers, relying instead on stethoscopes and [Sus-Phrine] injections. All these doctors are very busy and I have always been reluctant to ask if these things would help Aaron, especially since he cannot achieve a therapeutic level of theophylline without severe hyperactivity, crying jags and insomnia. How do I put these concerns into questions? I would like our doctor to "update," but where do I start?*

I suggest that parents who are in this type of a situation write a letter to the doctor detailing the problem. In all fairness to many good doctors out there, they are human and the routines of life can sneak up on them just like anyone else. Sometimes it takes a caring patient to remind a doctor gently that what he does in his office has a direct impact on the home. His response should indicate a willingness to explore the points raised in the letter. Under no circumstances should a parent of a patient be expected to sacrifice a child's free breathing by remaining loyal to a doctor. In fact, as the following letter attests, many mothers have felt the frustrating need to communicate their feelings to their doctors in a productive manner.

A Mother's Letter

> *See if you recognize the following scenario: you are awakened in the middle of the night to face the total panic of a young child who can't breathe. You think he may have croup but you're not sure. Clearly, you've got to do something or one of these noisy breaths may be his last. You remain calm, you*

quickly give him some medicine, you sit with him in the steamy bathroom, you coo him into relaxation and finally the situation is under control. You tuck him back into his bed and you return to yours, only to lie awake the rest of the night and tiptoe quietly into his room several times to reassure yourself.

The next morning he seems okay, but it was a frightening experience for you both, so you call the pediatrician for an appointment . . . You're full of concern and wiped out from loss of sleep. You rearrange your schedule and trek off to the doctor's office. When it's your turn, you explain the situation, the doctor does a quick examination and because there is no apparent infection and the child's lungs sound clear at the moment, the doctor looks at you as if you are imagining things and pronounces the child to be in perfect health. You are quickly ushered out of his office and presented with a bill. So, you go home only to experience a repeat performance later that night.

Sound familiar? I've been there. If you have, too, I hope it didn't take too many of these real life nightmares before you wound up in the office of an asthma specialist as I did.

I am the mother of two asthmatic children, so I'm no stranger to doctors' waiting rooms. There are a few things I'd like to get off my chest, so what follows is an open letter to my children's doctor.

> *Dear Asthma Doctor:*
>
> *I love my children and I am totally dedicated to my homemaking and mothering career. I am committed to see that they are happy, healthy and develop to their fullest potential. One of my children has a problem right now, and I'm here because I need your help. As I see it, you and I are about to become a team. Our goal is to make this child as healthy as possible. You'll be the*

coach who sends in the plays from the sideline, and I'll be the quarterback who sees that the plays are executed properly. We may find that some of the plays will be more successful than others and we may have to react to some blitzes during the course of the game, but I feel confident that we will achieve our goal.

Here then, is a game plan for success.

1. Respect me. I may look pretty disheveled at the moment. I'm worried, and chances are I haven't had much sleep for at least the past few nights. You see, I've been up with my sick child (your patient). No matter what my background is or how much education I've had, I hold a very important position—I am the mother of this child.

2. Listen to me. I know you have spent years studying and practicing medicine, that's why I've come to you. But I know my child. I know when there's something wrong. So listen through your stethoscope, but before you make a judgment, put it away and listen to me. What I can tell you is at least as important as what it can.

3. Educate me. Answer my questions, but don't limit yourself to that. Realize that asthma and allergy are things that I knew nothing about until my child first began to have problems. I may be so overwhelmed by what you're telling me that I don't know what questions to ask! But I am the one who will be caring for your patient. I will be carrying out your instructions and apprising you of further developments. I've had no special preparation for this position, and if I'm to do my job well, I need some on-the-job training. I need to have a working understanding of what's going on in my child's body and what to expect from the medications you are instructing me to administer.

4. Let me know what you expect of me. You will direct the course of treatment in this child's case. You need to make clear the direction you plan to take—the tests, medications or methods of treatment you plan to pursue and what about follow-up? As the child grows, there are many variables—sensitivities change, dosages of medications need to be adjusted, etc.—I need to know exactly what is expected of me in administering medication to my child. The pharmacist types instructions for dispensing the medicine, but I need to know about possible side effects, what results are expected and how long before I should expect to see them. Some drugs act immediately and some take several days to reach a therapeutic level—I need to know what should be happening and when to report back to you if it's not.

5. Support me. Please realize that it's not only the asthmatic child who suffers. I am the one who has to deal with the panic when he can't breathe. (I'm just as scared as he is, but it's up to me to calm him down.) I'm the one who is on the brink of exhaustion from countless nights of lost sleep. The patient can sleep late the next day or take a nap, but I have my normal responsibilities to carry out. I can't tell you how many nights I've sat up and listened to my children wheeze and cough while they sleep right through it. Many times I've had to wake them up to give them medicine. I'm the "meanie" who has to take them for weekly shots, make them take nasty-tasting medicines and enforce the restrictions they must live with. I'm the one who worries because I feel there must be something more I can do to make them comfortable, but I don't know what it is.

Trying to keep a child's asthma under control is like trying to walk a tightrope. Offer me a net! *Make me aware of organizations and publications that offer moral support for people in my position. Sometimes I just need somebody to talk to who understands what life with an asthmatic is like. I don't want to bother you or your staff, but I need a place to turn. I have been fortunate enough to "luck into" knowledge about a few helpful resources, but I feel that providing the families of your young patients with an awareness of available support is one of your basic responsibilities.*

Respectfully yours,
Debbie Scherrer

What is encouraging is that we do receive mail expressing satisfaction with doctors, too:

My five-year-old twin boys have recently been diagnosed as having asthma. We have gone through three hospitalizations within the last six months but thanks to a knowledgeable and concerned allergist, we have been able to avoid that recently.

* * *

Michael's asthma is very difficult to control. We went from doctor to doctor until I finally called the Lung Line in Denver. (See Resources section.) They gave me the name of a Dr. Weinstein, who trained at their hospital. He was finally able to balance medication and control and taught me how to make the necessary adjustments for Michael's asthma. His office is an hour and a half trip for us. However, it has been worth every minute.

When should you seek a second opinion from another doctor? If your child is hospitalized more than three times a year, if your doctor proclaims he is doing his best and your child is still not responding properly, if asthma claims more of your life than you have to give, seek a second opinion. To ensure you get your money's worth from the second doctor, do your homework first. Select this doctor carefully and send records, charts and test results to the doctor in advance of your visit and then call to confirm that the information was received. Getting a second opinion doesn't mean you don't trust your primary doctor or that you don't respect her. It means you are doing the very best you can for your child.

The important thing to remember is never to settle for mediocrity. Never stop looking for solutions to your child's asthma. There is someone out there who is willing and able to help you and your child. Never give up. There are medical solutions to your child's physical problems.

As this mom in Michigan wrote, *keep looking* until you find the right doctor for your child:

> *Currently, my two-and-a-half-year-old son is being treated by his fourth doctor, an asthma/allergy specialist. His first doctor misdiagnosed asthma, which began when my son was six weeks old. He also overlooked a total bowel blockage at eight weeks old. His second doctor said that at age fourteen months, Brett would outgrow the chronic ear infections and was diagnosed as "having the tendency to wheeze." When Brett became more sickly with repeated bouts of pneumonia and "wheezing," a ruptured eardrum and repeated ear infections and I made mention of my concern, I was told, "Brett is no more sick than any other child."*
>
> *This led to doctor number three and finally the good*

> *Lord gave me wisdom to seek a lung specialist on my own. After two years of misdiagnosed illness I was losing faith in pediatricians. However, this time, a correct diagnosis was made of chronic asthma with allergies. A new treatment plan has been started and Brett is so much better now.*
>
> *Through all of this I have learned that as a mother, I know my child better than any doctor. I have had doctors treat me as if I were a fool fabricating my child's illnesses or problems. We are the only source of communication for our preschool-age children. Search for that doctor who will listen, believe and help you. Your child's life is worth the price you pay for proper care.*

Doctors who are skilled in asthma and allergy management provide the most important part of your child's health care, *the management plan.* Without this, no child with asthma breathes very easily.

QUACKERY

Now you know how to find a good doctor. But you should also learn to recognize those who follow practices which may not have any scientific or medical basis.

When you and I are hurting, we look for answers, answers which may never come unless we go looking in the right places. Sometimes, because our resources are limited or our doctors are not current on contemporary asthma management practices, we search in vain. Our frustrations mount as we watch our children suffer. The longer asthma rages out of

OFFICE VISIT

Make the most of each office visit. It is the most valuable opportunity you have to learn about your child's asthma. Too often we are distracted and either do not understand or forget some of what the doctor tells us, or some of the questions we have been meaning to ask may be forgotten in the pressure of the visit. Use this form to prepare for an office visit, writing down questions as they arise. Also use it to record each visit with your child's doctor—take notes and ask the doctor to read the form over before you leave, to ensure that you have an accurate understanding of information and instructions.

DATE OF VISIT _____ **Doctor's Name** _____

QUESTIONS AND CONCERNS (To be completed by parent prior to seeing the physician)

PHYSICAL EXAM (Record here any symptoms present or observations by your physician)

PROCEDURES, LAB TESTS, ETC.	**RESULTS**

NOTES CONCERNING DOCTOR'S INSTRUCTIONS

Physician's Initials _____

control, the more vulnerable we become to those who would take our money but never provide relief.

I don't expect doctors to perform overnight miracles; however, if a doctor keeps abreast of the latest medical technology and teaches patients appropriate self-management skills, his patients are going to benefit.

Many times, when we go from doctor to doctor in search of answers we can live with, we begin to believe that we have exhausted all that medicine has to offer and that questionable methods of management are all that is left. We weigh our choices and wonder if it is indeed worth another try.

I have received many letters and calls from people who have explored "alternative forms" of medicine. A few of these people were enthusiastic about the treatment they received and indeed a few of them do seem to have experienced genuine relief. Most people, however, give humble, somber accounts of spending enormous sums of money for consultant fees, special diets and vitamins and massages. Their only objective in sharing their humiliation is to prevent others from walking down the same path.

Yes, there are good doctors and there are bad ones. However, we must always be aware that sometimes we are so desperate for freedom from asthma that our sense of judgment is distorted. Sometimes the quack is so convincing that you are willing to risk everything. How do we avoid the bad ones long enough to find the good ones?

- *Look for a track record of successful management.* A satisfied customer who has stayed satisfied for a long time is your first clue that the services provided will be worth the money.

- *Call your local Better Business Bureau, local Medical Society, and AMA (American Medical Association).* See if any grievances have been lodged against the person. If so, take your money elsewhere.

- *What qualifies this person to provide the services he claims will control asthma?* What medical degrees has the person earned? Is this person certified by the medical board of his specialty and is the specialty one that is recognized by the American Medical Association? Asthma is a medical problem with medical answers. Not all asthma requires medications all the time but all asthma does require someone who understands the physiology of the disease, how to improve the quality of life for patients and what to do in case of emergency. Some quacks have been known to create the emergencies by their medical incompetence.

- *If the practitioner promises a cure, write or call any of the organizations listed in the Resource section of this book and see if they know anything about this cure.* Scientists, doctors and researchers are looking for a cure but they have not found one as yet. Until then, management and control are our best allies.

- *Check your health insurance policy for coverage information.* It is always a good idea to do this before making an appointment with any doctor. Not all doctors participate in all insurance plans. If your insurance coverage does not include the services of a doctor you have chosen, find out why and discuss this in advance of your appointment.

  Also, be aware that many proponents of questionable practices want all their money up front. That is because insurance companies don't pay insurance claims to those who provide questionable services. If you don't pay, they don't get paid at all.

• *Do not be fooled by rigid rules.* Those who practice quackery rarely have scientific data to support their claims.
Their treatment plans often include impossibly rigid rules,
exotic diets and complicated instructions. This is what I
call their "fail-safe insurance plan." When the treatment
fails, the provider blames "parental and patient noncom-
pliance." Most parents become even more discouraged following an experience with a quack. They believe that all
hope for control has been exhausted. Remember that controlled asthma does not consume life—it provides the freedom to live it.

Consider carefully how you spend your money and whom
to trust to help your children. Be decisive. Learn as much
about the disease and methods of control as you can. Do not
believe the lie that asthma can be cured, yet. Control of
asthma is the next best thing, and control *is* possible. Never
stop working toward it and a better day will be coming.

PAYING FOR HEALTH CARE

While you are thinking about finding a good doctor (if you
don't already have one), be thinking about how you are going
to pay for her services. Asthma out of control affects every
part of family life including finances. Getting asthma under
control costs money, sometimes lots of it, but once it is controlled, the costs do begin to subside or at least become more
predictable.

Parents' frustrations range from trying to obtain health insurance that pays for asthma to having an entire family of

asthmatics and not being able to afford to buy medicine except for whichever person is most sick.

One mother called me yesterday and said that four out of five members of her family have asthma and her husband's union insurance plan does not cover asthma except for the husband. They can afford medication only for whichever person is most sick. She understands that the way to overcome the asthma is to get it under control and keep it there but they can't afford the medication or the doctors' fees in order to gain control. They don't qualify for state aid because her husband makes a "decent" salary. What the state regulations don't consider is the percentage of the salary that goes to medications and treatment. It really doesn't matter how much money a person earns if he has to spend the majority of it on medications.

Where can parents turn for help? Health maintenance organizations are offered as group memberships usually through an employer, though some HMO's also accept individual members. Group health plans are growing in popular-

A $70,000 BILL

Our two-year-old son started life two months before schedule and in respiratory arrest. He has had many problems since then, one of which is asthma. He takes many medications three times a day. He is often out of control. His doctors now suggest allergy testing, so maybe we will learn something new that might help. We feel so helpless and inadequate as we watch our baby suffer. Our lifestyle has been greatly affected. Medical bills and prescriptions for him are over $70,000 at this point and if it weren't for our insurance, we feel we would have lost everything. I try to keep faith that someday things will get better. I just look at my beautiful son and say, "I love you very much." He makes it all worthwhile. His doctors all work together to get rid of this thing called asthma.—Mother in Brazoria, Texas

ity. For a fixed amount of money each month, you prepay your dental, medical and optical expenses. Many times prescriptions are included in the package. Most HMO's pay for medical treatment but not for tools of the trade, such as peak flow meters and nebulizers.

In looking for a HMO type of plan, examine the fine print. Make sure the primary care physician has both the authority and the inclination to make referrals to specialists if necessary. Interview prospective pediatricians, allergists, pulmonologists or internists to determine their responsiveness to the needs of the child with asthma.

If you are using a private insurance plan, find out what types of coverage it offers and make certain that asthma is covered. The coverage under traditional insurance plans varies. Some exclude asthma or any preexisting medical condition. In any case, the patient is usually responsible for a portion of the bill.

Many doctors program their patients to rely on emergency room services as opposed to teaching them self-management and prevention. As you will notice in the letter from the mother in Anaheim, crisis management drives the cost of asthma sky high. Crisis management requires increased hospitalizations, dependency on emergency room services and frequent use of expensive medications.

Until recently, crisis management of asthma was stan-

PRIVATE INSURANCE

My son has had mild asthma since he was about two years old. My husband and I never worried about it or learned much about it because he only had trouble a couple of times in two years when he got a cold and the doctor gave him Alupent.

Last year, he turned four and it was an eye-opening year for us. To make a long story short, our pediatrician had a "ho

dard fare. However, now that doctors are enabling their patients to control asthma daily, the high cost of asthma on an individual basis is coming down. Take our personal example with Brooke. I don't even know how many times she was hospitalized for asthma or how many trips to the emergency room we made in her first six years of life. I lost count. Ever since her asthma management plan was fine-tuned in April of 1985, she has not required even one hospitalization and has had only two emergency room visits— one of those was for multiple bee stings and the other was because I did not learn that Brooke was having problems breathing until six hours after her attack had started. (I was out shopping! How's that for a guilt trip.)

Not only has our asthma management plan kept us out of the hospital, it keeps us out of the doctor's office and active in life. Brooke sees her pediatrician for annual checkups and regular kid stuff like a

hum" attitude about asthma and we were too uninformed to know the difference. As a result, my son, Jon-Michael, ended up hospitalized for pneumonia complicated by asthma. That was last April. It was a very scary, confusing time. Since then, we've been to the ER twice more for shots, been to the doctor countless times and Jon-Michael (now five years old) is on both Theo-Dur and Alupent continuously.

One of our biggest challenges is financial. My husband is self-employed and we must purchase private insurance. Our Blue Cross insurance waived Jon-Michael's asthma when we purchased it three years ago. We thought nothing of it much because he never went to the doctor and had no problems with it. We had no idea it could get worse. Consequently, the problems of this year have caused us great financial hardship. Facing the prospect of another winter of expensive medicines, ER visits or hospitalizations is frightening. Because asthma is a preexisting condition, do others face these same problems? Are there any places we can turn? Any insurance companies that would cover my son? We applied to California Children's

Services but his asthma wasn't severe enough, yet. Surely we are not the only ones in the world with private insurance and asthma!—Mother in Anaheim, California

sore throat or jammed finger. She now goes to the allergist twice a year, mostly for management plan adjustments. When asthma flares do occur, if I feel uncomfortable about making a decision I call her doctor early enough in the flare for recommendations to be made over the phone. By keeping a daily diary and charting her peak flow meter readings, we prevent the need for crisis intervention.

The emergency room is the correct place to go if the asthma management plan breaks down. However, emergency rooms are equipped to save lives, not control asthma. It makes no sense that most insurance companies that do cover asthma will pay indefinitely for crisis management of the disease but ignore the very preventive services which can help them reduce their costs. This situation is particularly descriptive of health care options available through government agencies for the poor, but it is also typical of some "high option" policies provided through private insurers.

I wonder what would happen if insurance companies covered a specified number of regularly scheduled office visits and a specific number of unscheduled office visits and set a limit on the number of emergency room visits it would cover each year. I believe the quality of life for those with asthma would improve. I also believe that asthma-related health costs would decrease for those doctors and their patients who take asthma more seriously.

It is not only doctors and parents who need to keep abreast of modern means of controlling asthma. A reassessment by the health insurance industry is certainly long overdue.

CHAPTER 5

WHAT PARENTS NEED TO KNOW ABOUT MEDICATIONS, ALLERGY TESTS, AND IMMUNOTHERAPY

MEDICATIONS AND ALLERGY THERAPY MAKE up but one piece of the jigsaw puzzle of asthma management. Asthma and allergy medications do not cure asthma and allergies. They can only address the symptoms, and at this writing there is no single medication that controls asthma or allergy symptoms in all people all the time.

Parents should understand the primary, intended functions of the medications and therapies the doctor prescribes.

In the following sections, Martha Vetter White, M.D., pediatric allergist at National Institutes of Health, Bethesda, Maryland, and also the medical editor of *MA Report,* provides this practical approach to understanding medications and therapies used in asthma-management plans today:

> *There are three ways to approach the treatment of asthma and other allergic diseases. The first is to determine your triggers and avoid them. This is by far the most effective approach. Total avoidance is certainly possible for food and animal allergic persons. Dust exposure can be markedly reduced by air filtration, bedroom simplifications and frequent housecleaning. The entrance of outside allergens into the home can also be substantially reduced by air-filtration and air-conditioning systems. All of these techniques help considerably and should be seriously pursued by any patient with significant allergic symptoms. Clearly, if all triggers could be avoided, there would be no symptoms and no need for medications.*
>
> *Unfortunately it is frequently impossible to avoid all allergens and other triggers. When symptoms occur despite good avoidance techniques, medications (the second approach) are prescribed.*
>
> *Some medications act by both preventing pathologic changes (the body's abnormal reaction to triggers) which lead to symptoms and by reversing existing symptoms. Examples of these medications are theophylline products and beta adrenergic bronchodilators (adrenaline-like medicines) such as Alupent, Proventil, Ventolin or Brethaire. These medications can be used daily to prevent asthma or during an asthma attack to reverse symptoms.*

A second group of medications have little, if any, ability to prevent pathologic changes. This group includes antihistamines and decongestants used to treat nasal allergies and congestion from other, nonallergic causes. Examples of antihistamines include chlorpheniramine, the major ingredient in most over-the-counter preparations and many prescription antihistamines, terfenadine (Seldane), brompheniramine (Bromfed, Dimetapp) and others. Common decongestants include pseudoephedrine (Sudafed and others) and phenylpropanolamine (found in many combination antihistamine/decongestant preparations).

A third group of medications works by preventing pathology and has no ability to reverse symptoms. Cromolyn (Intal, Nasalcrom, Opticrom) is the only drug in this class approved for use in the United States. As you may have guessed, cromolyn can be very effective for preventing symptoms of asthma or hay fever when taken regularly, but is useless for reversing attacks already in progress.

Corticosteroids such as oral prednisone and inhaled preparations such as beclomethasone (Beconase, Vancenase), flunisolide (AeroBid), and triamcinolone (Azmacort) could fit into the first class described, but I've chosen to segregate this group of drugs because their mechanism of action is unique. Patients who have frequent asthma or hay fever symptoms also have inflammation in the lungs or nose which causes them to be more susceptible to their asthma or hay fever triggers. Corticosteroids prevent and reverse this inflammation, thus making the patient more resistant to his triggers. This takes time to accomplish, and the effects of oral steroids generally take six or more hours to be felt.

The third therapeutic approach available is immunotherapy (shot therapy). I generally use immunotherapy for patients with definite allergen-triggered asthma or hay fever who still experience significant symptoms despite good environmental control. Immunotherapy works by decreasing the body's sensitivity to allergens, thus increasing the minimal allergen exposure required to produce symptoms. It will not directly affect asthma induced by infections, exercise and other nonallergic triggers.

However, patients experiencing allergic asthma attacks tend to be more reactive to other asthma triggers than when they're not already wheezing. Therefore, immunotherapy, by inhibiting allergic asthma, will inhibit this increased reactivity to other triggers.

It takes about a year of weekly injections to work up to a full dose of immunotherapy and the benefits are usually not seen until this time. Shots can then be given anywhere from weekly to monthly, depending on the response of the patient, and should be continued for three to five years. Once shots are stopped, benefits usually continue for a few years but then symptoms gradually begin to recur. At this point shots can be started again. Immunotherapy is quite useful for treating allergic asthma and hay fever but is of no benefit in the treatment of nonallergic asthma. The decision on whether to start shots is personal and depends on the relative frequency and severity of symptoms and the number of medications being taken, balanced against the initial expense and inconvenience of weekly office visits.

INSIDE THE MEDICINE CABINET

There is more to medicating our children than popping pills and pouring syrups down their throats. The medicines we give our children come in many forms; some to be inhaled, sprayed, rubbed in, swallowed or applied, one drop at a time. Medications come in syrups, sprays, pills, capsules, vials, powders, inhalers and drops. Some taste good and others taste horrible. Depending on the patient, the propellants, binders, dyes and even the chemistry of the medication itself can sometimes produce such negative side effects as mouth sores, nasal burning sensations, hyperactivity and stomach pain, to name just a few.

When we take our children to the doctor, I believe we are all looking for a quick fix. We want a pill that will make everything better. And when we come away with a dozen prescriptions for medicines we really don't fully understand, and then we see what a hassle it is to give them to a child who doesn't want to take them, we sometimes become disillusioned. We begin to feel trapped by the very tools which are a vital part of freeing us from asthma's tyranny.

Parents need to understand the characteristics, potential benefits and side effects of each of the medications their child is taking. They need to know when it is appropriate to use or taper off each medication, and what their interactions are with over-the-counter medications their child may be using.

None of this happens overnight. Parents don't become instant pharmacists simply because they give their children pills. However, your goal should be to understand the medications your child is using and to work with your doctor to fine-tune the asthma management plan as needed to avoid medication side effects.

I know parents who say, "Asthma means my child either doesn't breathe or he is wired up on drugs. It's one or the other. So when she gets bad enough, I'll start the medicine. But not a minute before."

Optimal asthma management is not trading one evil for another. The longer you wait to treat an attack of asthma, the more medications will be required to halt it. This child can't possibly function normally, because she is either struggling to breathe or suffering from medication side effects. This also describes the heartbreak of crisis management of asthma, a very dangerous flirtation with a potentially fatal outcome.

When a doctor prescribes a new medication or adjusts any which are currently part of your asthma-management plan, you should ask the following questions (if the doctor has not already answered them):

- What is the intended function of the medication?
- How quickly should the medication act?
- What is the appropriate action to take if the medication fails to deliver the expected results within the specified time allotted?
- What are the potential side effects of the medication?
- What response should be made to those side effects if they should occur?
- Under which circumstances should the medication be administered?

Many times those answers are provided by the doctor's nurse and through medication handout sheets.

With answers to these questions, parents will be able to

help determine the effectiveness of their children's treatment plan and communicate important information to their doctor.

The Medication Plan form will help you keep your doctor's instructions straight. Make a copy, and complete it with the help of your doctor. It should be revised each time an adjustment is made in your asthma-management plan. When asthma symptoms arise, act quickly according to your predetermined plan, since asthma flares are easily reversed in the early stages and are far more difficult to reverse if allowed to progress.

The information below, reprinted from *The Asthma Organizer,* should help you better understand the practical aspects of medications that your child's doctor may prescribe.

BETA-ADRENERGIC BRONCHODILATORS

Action

Beta adrenergics are very fast-acting bronchodilators that are related to adrenaline. These medications open the airways by relaxing the smooth muscles that surround the air tubes.

Administration

This class of medications comes in a variety of forms with different routes of administration. Some types are swallowed in the form of a liquid or tablet, some are inhaled via a metered-dose inhaler or nebulizer and some are injected. Notes concerning each form of administration are below.

Side Effects

Potential side effects of beta adrenergics include shakiness, jitteriness, pallor, nervousness, rapid heartbeat, nausea and

M E D I C A T I O N   P L A N
(Courtesy of *The Asthma Organizer)*

Name of Medication   Administration—dosage, times, etc.

FIRST-LINE MEDICATION(S) To begin at the first sign of
asthma symptoms or for routine use on a daily basis

BACKUP PLAN To be used if asthma symptoms persist in spite
of first-line medication(s)

CALL PROMPTLY WHEN:

DOCTOR'S NAME:

DATE:

vomiting. Dryness or irritation of the mouth or throat associated with inhaler use can be avoided by rinsing the mouth with water and swallowing a few sips after using the inhaler. More severe side effects to be reported to your doctor are chest pain, irregular, pounding heartbeat, severe headache or dizziness, extreme nausea or vomiting.

There are a number of brands of drugs in this classification. Some of these include: Alupent, Brethaire, Bronkometer, MaxAir, Proventil, Tornalate, and Ventolin. Notify your doctor if the medication you are using does not provide desired results or causes uncomfortable side effects. It is possible that another bronchodilating medication may work more effectively.

Oral Beta-Adrenergic Bronchodilators

Liquids or tablets begin to act within thirty minutes and last as long as four to six hours.

Many young children begin with the oral method of delivery and as they grow older progress to the inhaled route, which generally produces fewer side effects.

Beta-Adrenergic Bronchodilators via Metered-Dose Inhaler

Begin to work within fifteen minutes and last as long as four to six hours.

Inhalers are effective only if the proper technique is employed. Correct positioning and proper timing are crucial. Holding chambers called spacers facilitate the use of inhalers. Some common spacers are InspirEase, AeroChamber and InhalAid. (See Chapter 6.)

If your doctor prescribes two inhalations, wait five to ten minutes between puffs to allow the first one to open the airways for better penetration by the second. Similarly, if you also use an inhaled steroid or cromolyn at the same time, use the bronchodilating inhaler first.

Overuse of the inhaler can cause very serious complications. *Do not* use more frequently than prescribed. If you feel the need to use the inhaler again before it is time for the next dose, this is a sign that your child's asthma is out of control and you should discuss this with your doctor.

The use of a bronchodilating inhaler twenty minutes before strenuous exercise prevents exercise-induced asthma in many patients.

Beta-Adrenergic Bronchodilators via Nebulizer

Medications delivered by compressor-driven nebulizer work in the same manner as those taken by metered-dose inhaler. Nebulizers are particularly beneficial for infants and children who are too young to master the inhaler.

They are also useful for older children and adult patients with moderate to severe asthma because they deliver medications more effectively

WHAT YOU CAN DO NOW

You can help ensure that your child's asthma attacks are treated early by recognizing the early signs of an oncoming asthma attack and treating at that point. Keep a daily symptom diary (such as the one found in *The Asthma Organizer,* see Resources), paying attention to cough, chest tightness, nasal symptoms, sleep disturbances, shortness of breath, wheezing and energy level. Discuss the findings with your doctor and try to pinpoint the earliest symptoms in an attack. Maybe your child starts coughing the day before, or maybe every time he plays soccer when he's coughing, he comes in wheezing. Each child has his own pattern. Let the flow meter readings help you.

Have your doctor outline a plan for treating attacks early and be sure you understand what to use, when and how much. Also, be sure you understand how fast the medications should work. If things aren't improving as expected, you

and produce a more significant result when lung function is greatly impaired.

Beta-Adrenergic Bronchodilators via Injection

Injected adrenaline or epinephrine (names are interchangeable) is used in the doctor's office or emergency room for an acute asthma attack. It works immediately but is a very short-acting medication, lasting only twenty minutes. Sus-Phrine is a longer-acting form of injected adrenaline, lasting six hours.

should consult with your doctor to see if a change in medications or an office emergency room visit is necessary. *Call early. Don't wait for the attack to become severe.*

If you think a medication is causing undesirable side effects, call your doctor. Some patients stop medications on their own because of side effects. This is sometimes the right thing to do, but often the wrong medication is stopped out of ignorance. Sometimes the "side effect" has nothing to do with the medication stopped, and the parent denies the child a valuable form of treatment.

—Martha V. White, M.D.

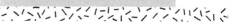

CROMOLYN

Action

Cromolyn is thought to stabilize the mast cell, preventing the release of its mediators, such as histamine, that lead to an asthma flare. To state it more simply, the mast cell acts like a quarterback about to get sacked in an allergic reaction. It carries the allergic antibody on it and, when exposed to a substance to which the person is allergic, it throws out granules containing histamine and other chemicals. The body responds to these chemicals with a chain of reactions resulting in asthma and other allergy symptoms. Cromolyn is thought to prevent the mast cell from throwing out its granules, thus preventing the allergic reaction.

Administration

Intal, the only brand name of cromolyn for the lungs currently being produced, comes in three forms: 1) the powder-filled capsule, which is used with an inhaler (Spinhaler); 2) metered-dose inhaler; and 3) nebulizer solution to be used with a compressor-driven nebulizer. A nasal form (Nasalcrom) and eyedrop form (Opticrom) are also available for those who suffer with hay fever.

Side Effects

Cromolyn is a safe medication used in the treatment of asthma. The Spinhaler may induce coughing or wheezing in some users, but these side effects are generally not found when Intal is delivered via the metered-dose inhaler or nebulizer. These methods of delivery sometimes leave a bad taste in the mouth, which can be avoided by rinsing the mouth and drinking a few sips of water after the inhalation.

Notes

This is a preventive medication and will provide no relief during an asthma attack. Check with your doctor regarding use during an asthma episode.

Since cromolyn is a preventive medication, it may be difficult for the patient to determine if it is providing any benefit. Additionally, it may take as long as four weeks of continuous use to reach effectiveness.

Intal must reach deep into the airways for full effectiveness. Your doctor may tell you to use a beta-adrenergic bronchodilator five minutes before using Intal to open the airways.

The use of Intal twenty minutes before strenuous exercise prevents exercise-induced asthma in many patients.

Nebulizers make it possible for infants to use this medication.

THEOPHYLLINE

Action

Theophylline opens the airways by relaxing the smooth muscles that surround the air tubes. Recent investigations also ascribe an anti-inflammatory action to theophylline.

Administration

It is important to follow the doctor's instructions for administration closely. Give carefully measured doses as close as possible to the prescribed time. It is best to take theophylline with some food rather than on an empty stomach.

There are many brand names of theophylline with different forms ranging from rapid-absorption preparations to long-acting preparations. If your theophylline preparation is in *tablet* form it must be swallowed, not chewed, at the designated times. The *capsule* form of theophylline may be swallowed, or for younger children the contents can be sprinkled on a small amount of sweet food such as applesauce, jelly or honey to disguise its bitter taste. The *sprinkles* should be swallowed, not chewed, as chewing would release too much of the

DAILY DOSES

. . . After many hospitalizations, we have discovered that Timmy is a rapid metabolizer of theophylline and we have had a difficult time controlling his attacks without the effects of overmedication. At the present, he is on daily theophylline as well as nebulizer treatments three times a day. We have especially found it very difficult with Timmy's schooling. He is currently enrolled in private school where they have been very cooperative in working with him.—Mother in Circleville, Ohio

time-release medication at once. Use a very small amount of food (one or two spoonfuls) to be sure that all the sprinkles are ingested, and not allowed to dissolve first. Do not mix with a hot food, which tends to dissolve the time-release sprinkles and release too much medication at once.

If you realize you've missed a dose *do not* attempt to make it up by doubling the next dose.

Some medications and other factors affect the way the body metabolizes theophylline. Therefore, if your child is taking theophylline, be sure your doctor is aware of *all* the other medications your child is taking. The antibiotic Erythromycin will cause the theophylline level to rise, as will Tagamet. While your child is taking these medications it will probably be necessary for your doctor to decrease his dosage of theophylline.

Side Effects

Potential side effects of theophylline include nausea, vomiting, stomach cramps, diarrhea, headache, increase in urination, muscle cramps, irregular heartbeat, shakiness or restlessness. Notify your doctor if your child experiences any of these side effects, as it may mean that the dosage should be adjusted. Mild side effects will often disappear after taking the medication for a while.

Notes

Chemically, theophylline is very closely related to caffeine and has the same stimulating effect. Consumption of caffeine-containing substances such as coffee, tea, cola drinks, cocoa and chocolate should be limited when taking theophylline.

Sustained-action theophylline preparations such as Theo-Dur and Slo-bid do not act immediately. It may take up to thirteen hours after the first dose for an effective blood level to be reached.

Parents and teachers may note changes in behavior patterns when a child is taking theophylline.

Blood Test

One way to determine accurately an individual's most effective dosage of theophylline is to check the serum level of theophylline in the blood. This simple blood test is done after a patient has been taking the medication long enough to attain a steady serum concentration. The usual therapeutic range is between 10 to 20 micrograms of theophylline per milliliter of blood serum. At levels lower than this the drug may or may not be as effective; at higher levels it may or may not be toxic and produce very undesirable side effects. Follow your doctor's instructions for scheduling this theophylline-level test.

STEROIDS

Action

Steroids (also called corticosteroids) decrease inflammation and mucus production, decrease hyperreactivity (twitchiness) of the airway and increase the effectiveness of other asthma medications.

Administration

Steroid use generally falls into two patterns, oral or inhaled. The administration of oral steroids is usually divided into three categories: burst, alternate morning and daily.

The most common use of oral steroids is a "pulse" or "burst" format. This short three- to seven-day course is designed to reduce swelling in the airways. If the physician determines that the need for bursts of steroids arises too frequently, the next step is usually alternate morning doses of the medication.

Once a person's asthma has been stabilized with a burst of steroids, the administration of alternate morning steroids (AMS) is often sufficient to control the asthma. This is a long-term step usually reserved for moderate to severe asthma. Many patients can receive treatment this way over an extended period of time without perceptible side effects.

It is of critical importance that the medication instructions be followed exactly when giving alternate morning steroids. If alternate morning steroids fail and the patient remains unstable, steroids may have to be administered daily. Fraught with side effects, this form of treatment is reserved for the most severely involved patients. This is not a common format.

The newest development in steroid therapy is their use in an inhaled form, now available as Beclovent, Vanceril, Azmacort, and AeroBid. The idea is to use the medication only on the area of need (in this case the interior of the airways), theoretically requiring a much smaller dose of steroids to reach the same level of stability. Because only a negligible amount of the medication is absorbed into the body, inhaled steroids can be used over the long term without the side effects associated with long term use of oral steroids.

It can take one to four weeks for inhaled steroids to reach effectiveness. Do not assume that the medication is not working and discontinue its use without first consulting your doctor.

Effectiveness of inhaled steroids is dependent upon how well the patient can use the inhalers. Therefore your doctor or his nurse should periodically check your child's inhaler technique.

Side Effects

The side effects of short-term doses or bursts of steroids do not usually appear unless the medication has been used daily for longer than two weeks. Short-term side effects can include an increased appetite, a feeling of well-being, fluid retention, and weight gain. Moodiness may be experienced when the steroid is stopped. Stomach upset, sometimes caused by this medication, can be reduced by taking it with some food.

The risk of developing side effects varies in proportion to the dosage of steroid and length of time taken. Use of an every-other-day dosing schedule reduces the risk of side effects. Steroids suppress the body's adrenal function, impairing its ability to respond to severe physical stress such as major injury or surgery. Other adverse effects usually associated with daily or higher doses of steroids are growth retardation in children, osteoporosis, cataracts, roundness of the face, development of facial hair, weight gain, elevation of blood sugar and blood pressure, muscle weakness, salt and fluid retention, acne, thinning of the skin, and mood changes.

The only side effect generally associated with inhaled steroids is an irritation or infection of the mouth or throat called thrush. Always gargle with water and swallow a few sips after each use. The use of a spacer will reduce the likelihood of a yeast infection, and will allow the medication to be delivered to the airways more effectively.

Notes

Long-term steroid use should never be stopped abruptly. Gradual tapering of the dose is necessary to prevent withdrawal symptoms such as muscle and joint achiness, fatigue, weakness, dizziness, and fever. *Never* discontinue steroid use without first consulting with your physician.

In case of severe injury or surgery, the physician must be made aware of present or recent steroid therapy. Steroid-dependent patients often wear a medical identification bracelet.

ANTICHOLINERGIC MEDICATIONS

Action

Anticholinergics are bronchodilators that are related to atropine. These bronchodilators are slower-acting than the beta-adrenergic (adrenaline-like) medications, taking about thirty to sixty minutes to peak, the effect of which lasts for four to six hours. Anticholinergics are also not as potent as the beta-adrenergic drugs. They have been useful, however, in treating excessive mucus or when components of bronchitis make up part of the disease. Anticholinergics prevent nerves in the airways from stimulating muscle contraction. These nerves can be activated by infections, inflammation, anxiety and psychic stress, and allergic reactions.

Administration

This class of medications comes as a metered dose inhaler (Atrovent). In addition, some physicians prefer to prescribe atropine for use in a nebulizer (see note about FDA approval on page xiii). Make sure you use this inhaler with your eyes closed. If the spray gets in your eyes, it will dilate them.

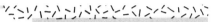

PARANOID

My son was diagnosed as having asthma last year due to allergies. He also has other allergy problems such as ear infections, headaches and nose problems.

I feel totally helpless. My medicine cabinet looks like a pharmacy. I have asthma pills, syrups, nose sprays, antihistamines, decongestants, and my doctor expects me to know when it is time to switch from one to another.

I cannot recognize an asthma problem. I cannot distinguish an asthma cough from a postnasal drip cough. As a result, I have become paranoid and I think my son is becoming a hypochondriac. My son is eight and has what the doctor calls mild asthma. I think this is why I have a hard time seeing these things even when he complains he can't breathe. I need help.—A mother from Brooklyn, New York.

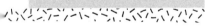

Side Effects

Potential side effects of anticholinergics include dry mouth, cough, headache and blurred vision. Irritation (but not dryness) of the mouth or throat associated with inhalation of anticholinergics can be avoided by rinsing the mouth with water and swallowing a few sips after using the inhaler. Another potential side effect is difficulty in urination, especially in older men.

MEDICATION MYTHS

Theophylline, an oral bronchodilator, causes learning disabilities.

Theophylline does *not cause* learning disabilities, but its side effects may make some children appear to have learning problems. The child may be more restless, nervous or irritable than usual. There is also evidence that *some* children taking theophylline may have greater problems with memory and concentration and in processing abstract concepts. The truth is, there is a great deal of misinformation and controversy surrounding this topic. Several studies are now examining theophylline's effect on learning and behavior.

Antihistamine and bronchodilators should not be used simultaneously.

At one time it was thought that the drying action of an antihistamine would interfere with the expected actions of bronchodilators. Recent studies show that this is rarely a problem, particularly with selective antihistamines now available.

To avoid unnecessary medications, wait to see if the attack goes away before treating your child.

Asthma is easier to prevent or halt than it is to treat!

THERAPIES ON THE HORIZON

Parents of asthmatic children for whom current medications and therapies are not working should take heart—advancements are coming down the road! For a look at current research, we turned again to Dr. White:

There are several exciting areas of ongoing research in the field of allergy. In the field of pharmacology, most efforts are being applied toward improving classes of drugs currently in use in the United States. One of these improved drugs, terfenadine (Seldane) is a non-sedating antihistamine which has already been granted FDA approval for use in persons twelve and older, and is now available as a long-acting pill. The company that manu-

factures Seldane is currently developing a liquid form of the drug for use in children. This antihistamine has little or no effect on the brain and thus does not cause the sleepiness or hyperactivity associated with most other antihistamines. There are also several other long-acting non-sedating antihistamines including astemizol and loratidine being studied. These agents are at various stages in the approval process and probably will be available in the near future.

Another drug which is being studied in clinical trials in the United States is ketotifen, an oral antihistamine with additional action similar to cromolyn sodium (Intal, Nasalcrom and Opticrom). Ketotifen has been used in Europe to prevent asthma attacks for over a decade and is being studied in the United States both for prevention of asthma and for treatment of urticaria (hives). Its major advantage over cromolyn is that it can be taken twice a day orally and works systemically throughout the body. Its major disadvantage compared with cromolyn is that it can cause sleepiness in some patients. Ketotifen is available through research studies but is not yet approved for general use in the United States and probably won't be available for at least two to three years.

Several old favorites in our medication arsenal have just been released in new forms more convenient for children. Albuterol, a beta-adrenergic bronchodilator used by mouth or by inhalation to treat asthma, is now available for use in a nebulizer. This form is a distinct advantage over the unit-dose inhaler, which is more difficult to use effectively in small children. One pharmaceutical company which manufactures albuterol, Allen & Hanburys, recently came out with a powdered form

*of inhaled albuterol called Ventolin Rotacaps. The spe-
cial design of the inhaler provides an alternative for
those people who must use a spacer.*

*For those patients who have difficulty coordinating
use of the unit dose inhalers, a variety of spacers are
available, many in compact forms. These devices,
which fit on the mouthpiece of the inhaler, generally
are equipped with one-way valves at the mouth end of
the chamber and allow the patient to inhale the medication over two or more breaths.*

*Familiar nasal steroid sprays, Beconase and
Vancenase, have recently been approved for use in patients six years and older in a new, nonstinging aqueous
base. This will be welcome relief for those of you who
have struggled with the older, more irritating steroid
nasal sprays.*

*In the area of immunotherapy (shot therapy), exten-
sive work is being done by the FDA in conjunction with
manufacturers of allergen extracts to improve and stan-
dardize the extracts (concentrated allergen used with
skin testing and immunotherapy) that allergists have
available both for skin testing and for therapy. You may
have noticed if you've ever changed allergists that the
new allergist wants to repeat the skin tests and possibly
to alter the dose or ingredients of your child's immunotherapy. The reason is that until recently, there was
no standardization of allergenic extracts. That means
that a bottle of ragweed 10,000 PNU (the unit of
strength) made by one manufacturer may have been a
different strength, and may even have contained different components than a bottle of ragweed 10,000 PNU
manufactured by a different company. As a result, your
child may have tested negative to ragweed in one doc-*

tor's office and positive in another because of variability in potency of the extracts or because one extract may have lacked the component your child was allergic to. For the same reasons, many allergists were reluctant to continue the same immunotherapy prescription started by another doctor when they were using materials which were potentially of different potency and content compared with what the patient had previously received.

The system is still far from perfect. Cat and ragweed were among the first allergens available as standardized products, and the list is growing. The cost of standardization and the work involved are enormous, and thus it's a slow process. But many years down the road, we can look forward to complete standardization of all allergenic products. This should improve safety while lowering costs by reducing the incidence of both repeat skin testing and the necessity for a new allergist to start different immunotherapy.

Also along the lines of immunotherapy, researchers are working on improved chemical forms of allergen extracts designed to decrease the time required to achieve the maximal dose of immunotherapy while reducing the risk of serious side effects. There are several different forms being studied, all at different stages in the FDA review process. As yet, none has received approval for use in the United States. Once approved, the new technology will probably be gradually applied to the various different allergens available for immunotherapy. Thus I suspect it will be a long time before this form of immunotherapy is widely available.

One of the most exciting areas of ongoing allergy research deals with controlling how much IgE (antibodies which are absolutely essential for allergic reactions to occur, and to which allergens attach in the bloodstream) is made by the body. Doctors in several medical centers throughout the country are discovering how various cells in the blood alter the production of IgE by sending special molecules to control or regulate IgE production. The hope is that if one could decrease the amount of IgE made by the body, one might be able to prevent persons with allergic potential from becoming sensitized to new allergens. Unfortunately, once formed, IgE remains in the body for long periods of time (probably years). Thus control of IgE production would probably not cure existing allergies but could prevent the development of new allergens and might prevent babies from becoming allergic children.

HOW TO HELP YOUR CHILD LEARN HOW TO SWALLOW PILLS AND TAKE OTHERWISE FOUL-TASTING MEDICINES

Now that you've been introduced to the technical side of asthma medications, you have to get them into your child's system. For some parents, this job is a kicker, and I do mean *kicker.*

Always make sure you understand your doctor's instructions before medicating your child. When dispensing medications, use exact measures. Don't use soup spoons or other tableware.

Infants can be especially squirmy and strong-willed if they don't want to take medicine. Many times parents must resort to creative means of medicating their tiny ones. One helpful trick is to purchase, at any drugstore pharmacy, a special liquid-medicine dispenser which looks like a syringe without the needle. Fill the dispenser to the appropriate level and slowly squirt the medication on the back of your baby's tongue or toward the back of the inside of the baby's cheek.

Some babies are adept at spitting a good portion of the medication back out once we think it's been swallowed. For those babies there is a medicine dispenser that is fitted with a baby bottle nipple at the top. The sucking reflex is immediate when the nipple is placed in the baby's mouth and before the baby can think about it or taste it, the medicine is gone.

There are some babies who resist all forms of trickery. When this happens you must resort to "brute force." Remember, it is extremely important for your baby to get the amount of medicine your doctor has prescribed. Your baby will forgive you for the momentary discomfort of being held down, and brute force really isn't all that traumatic in the first place. Here's how you *use* it. If you hold the baby's nose, he or she will eventually (usually immediately) open his mouth. Use a syringe suited for dispensing medications and squirt the medicine slowly onto the back of the baby's tongue. Don't let go of the nose until the baby has swallowed. Hopefully, that will be the last you will see of the medicine. Thankfully, most of the medications are now flavored and therefore easier for your baby to swallow.

Medications can be easier or can be even more difficult to administer to our children as they grow older. This simply means parents need to be more creative. Some asthma medications come in capsules that are designed to be broken and sprinkled on foods. However, some children don't like the taste and texture of the medication once the capsules are broken. Try sprinkling the medication on some of these treats: applesauce, Jell-O, Cool Whip, honey, jelly or pudding. However, avoid using caffeine-containing foods when giving theophylline medications.

If these tactics don't work, you could always try honesty and admit to your child that you know that medicine sometimes tastes pretty yucky. Encourage the child to be a big boy or girl and swallow a spoonful of the medicine mixed with the treat and follow it by a drink of fruit juice or a cookie. Praise obedience and a good attitude.

Motivate your child by a system of rewards (these are different from bribes; they are earned). Allow your child to place a sticker in a booklet every time he takes his medication. When he earns ten (or whatever number you choose) stickers, he can choose from a list of treats. Those treats might include staying up late one night to watch a favorite television show (will he need a nap that day?), having a friend come over to play or making cookies.

Swallowing pills can be very difficult for some children. We still tease our oldest son, Michael, because he was thirteen before he could swallow a pill. Before that we tried every trick in the book and he simply could not swallow anything he could not chew first! In *Pediatric Parents* (which credited the material to the July 1987 issue of *Medical Tribune*), I read about a trick that helps children forget they are swallowing a pill. Swallowing has two parts—thinking and reflex. If your child can be distracted, the reflex part takes over and the pill goes down easily. The pop-bottle method, as described by Dr. Joseph Fowler of the University of Louisville, uses the reflex part of swallowing: Have your child put the pill in her mouth and then put her lips tightly around the open end of a pop bottle. She should suck the liquid out of the pop bottle. The sucking motion will automatically cause the pill to go down.

Mary Beth at the Lung Line at the National Jewish Center for Immunology and Respiratory Medicine says: "Children should be able to swallow pills by age seven. If they cannot swallow pills by this age, they will probably always have difficulty with pills. At age two, parents can start teaching their children to swallow pills using glycerin capsules [fake pills]. Their gelatin coating makes it easier for children to swallow."

Some parents are able to encourage their toddlers to swallow pills by making a game of it, placing the pill on the back of the child's tongue and having the child swish it down with drink from a bottle. Some children find it easier to swallow pills when they sip the drink through a straw. A few parents have found great success using the small boxed fruit drinks to wash the pills down the throat.

Mary Beth also uses an "alligator spoon" to encourage her daughter to take medicines. You pour the medicine in the alligator's mouth to measure the correct amount and then the alligator "pours" the medicine into your child's mouth!

If your child is extremely reluctant to take pills, once again appeal to his or her sense of logic. Explain that a pill goes down more quickly and with less taste than a liquid. But children who are extremely reluctant to switch from liquids to pills should not be forced to do so unless there is no other choice.

And finally, this word from Dr. Bob Lanier in Fort Worth, Texas: "Capsules float and pills sink. Put a capsule on the tongue, take a drink and lean forward to swallow. Put a pill on the tongue and drink rapidly from a small-mouthed bottle —not a glass. The sucking negates the gag reflex. You can swallow even big pills this way."

ALLERGY TESTING

Allergy testing helps to determine what is affecting the child. Allergy testing today is usually (not always) done by pricking the skin and placing a drop of antigen (the substance to which your child is suspected of having an allergy) at the prick site. These prick sites are watched for signs of reaction. The reaction usually looks like a tiny red bump. The size of the bumps is usually proportional to the degree of allergy.

Allergy testing is usually done on the child's back or arms. The doctor may need to perform just a few tests, one little prick at a time, or may use a device which pricks the skin in multiple places at one time.

Many parents feel that the testing is far too traumatic to justify since no one is sure if any subsequent immunotherapy is going to be helpful. Although allergy testing is not pleasant, neither is it a form of medieval torture. Some children have a fear of needles, laboratories and doctors' offices and are therefore harder to test, but most children get through the procedure quite well. Often we parents suffer more than our children.

There are three basic options for treating allergy—avoidance, medication and immunization (allergy shots). Immunization is a method of reprogramming the immune system to react less violently. Children are candidates for allergy shots if they have unavoidable problems in spite of reasonble avoidance and medication.

If allergy shots are recommended after consultation, children may show some hesitation at first, but within time, they bounce right in for their shot without any complaints.

Parents must also understand that allergy testing can provide valuable information, but it is not foolproof. One such area concerns allergy testing for foods.

Though allergy testing for foods is not 100 percent accurate, it gives us a list of suspected culprits and an opportunity to remove them. Many times, in an effort to end their child's suffering, parents put them on severe diets or unjustly withhold too many foods hoping to discover just the right healthy balance. Allergy testing for foods provides clues that allow the parent and doctor to remove only those foods which are truly suspect. Once the child is stable for a period of time to be determined by the doctor, parents can begin to reintroduce the foods one at a time (also with instructions from your doctor) and watch for possible signs of allergy.

Remember: Allergy testing provides information that, when combined with other evidence and a medical history, your doctor will use to develop an asthma and allergy management plan which may or may not include allergy shots.

PREPARING YOUR CHILD FOR ALLERGY TESTING AND IMMUNOTHERAPY

In Chapter 1, I told you about my experiences with Brooke, who was eighteen months old when she was tested. We prepared Brooke for the testing at home by telling her we were going to see a special doctor who was going to try to help us make her asthma get better. We told her he was going to have to put special medicine on her back and that it would hurt but not for very long. We explained that I would hold her and she could squeeze me and she could even cry if she wanted to but she could not move around because that would hurt very much and would spoil the test. Then the doctor would have to do it all over again. Because of her young age, we prepared her one more time at the doctor's office, but this time when I explained it I added a little incentive to reward good behavior. I had brought along her most favorite treats—a lollipop and lipstick.

I was pregnant with Brooke's little brother at the time so when she sat on my lap with her arms wrapped around my expanded waist, her little back was exposed just right. The doctor used a device which injected ten test sites at once and four times he pressed the device on her back. Four times she let out a yell and squeezed me tight but she never moved. When she hopped off my lap the first thing she requested was her lipstick and after I applied it she went racing down the hall to tell her daddy about what the doctor had done to her back. One month later, we had another testing session for foods. This time there were no objections expressed by Brooke even at her tender age.

Some children have an irrational fear of doctors, shots and testing. But if the procedure is expected to reveal valuable information, and you have made the decision to go through with it, prepare your child with explanations he can understand.

The greater your child's fear of testing procedures, obviously, the more difficult it will be for him to submit to the testing. Gear your explanations to your child's ability to comprehend. There is no need to describe the size or number of the needles.

Incentives, not bribes, can help children who remain fearful over the hurdle. Incentives are those rewards which are earned for an appropriate behavior. Bribes are those things which children can turn around and use as a weapon on their parents if they are not careful.

Your doctor may instruct you not to use certain medications in the days prior to testing. Antihistamines, for example, should be avoided since they can interfere with the body's response and thereby give a false result on the test. Follow these instructions carefully. Many families have gone through the buildup of preparing the child for allergy tests only to reach the allergist's office and find out that the tests would have to be postponed because they had given the child an antihistamine.

Other medications that can interfere with skin testing results are cough and cold medicines that also contain antihistamine, medications like Tagamet (which, though not an antihistamine, can act as such), tranquilizers and sleeping pills. Be sure to provide a list of all prescription and over-the-counter medications to your doctor's nurse *before* your appointment.

If scheduled allergy injections are recommended, use the time spent in the waiting room constructively. To occupy young children, bring a book, or a plastic container full of little objects like blocks, a top, a yo-yo, a crayon and a tiny drawing tablet. A sewing craft such as cross-stitch or spool knitting can hold the interest of some young girls and boys. Helping a youngster sort a shoe box of baseball cards while waiting for the shot (and waiting for the shot to be checked before you can leave) makes the time seem to pass more quickly, is enriching to the mind, keeps your kids out of trouble and wards off otherwise inevitable complaints of boredom.

OTHER TESTS

You may also encounter tests to study the immune response in the blood. X-rays of the lungs are helpful in ruling out pneumonia, aspiration of foreign matter into the lungs and pneumothorax (a leak of air out of the lungs into the chest cavity, causing the lung to collapse). Sweat tests check for cystic fibrosis. Arterial blood gases are sometimes drawn in the emergency room to determine how well the lungs are oxygenating the blood and clearing the blood of carbon dioxide. A bronchoscopy may be needed if the doctor must retrieve foreign matter or mucus plugs from the lungs or if he requires a sampling of tissue from the bronchial lining in order to help make a diagnosis of other conditions.

Sometimes it seems as though there is too much work involved in understanding asthma. After all, the problem seems so simple. How can the solution be so complex? Whenever you begin to feel overwhelmed by the great magnitude of it all, take a break. Try to recapture a balanced perspective. Remind yourself that chronic asthma is a only a temporary problem if you persevere.

If you close your eyes, asthma won't go away. You have to face it squarely. Asthma and its control over your child and family will hang on to you only so long as you let it.

Do the best you can with the resources available to you. Take an active part in your child's asthma management plan. A better day is coming.

CHAPTER 6

TOOLS
OF
THE TRADE

USING THE RIGHT TOOLS IS IMPORTANT FOR ANY
job. Having the right tools for managing asthma can make a
big difference. There are specially designed tools that enable
our children to breathe more freely and live life more productively. Some of these tools monitor the openness of the
airways. Others assist in the delivery of medications. Some
are particularly helpful in preparing or cleaning the environment.

It is helpful to have a basic knowledge of the various tools of the trade that are available. Your doctor may recommend one or more of them to facilitate the asthma management plan. Product information is provided solely as an informational service in the Resource section of this book. Please discuss your desire or plans to purchase medical products with your doctor before you place your order. Inclusion of any product or service listed does not imply endorsement by Mothers of Asthmatics or me.

STETHOSCOPES

Our pediatrician introduced us to a stethoscope when Brooke was very small because I was constantly taking her to the doctor so she could listen to Brooke's chest. She taught me how to listen for and interpret wheezing sounds myself.

After putting the ear tips into my ears, I put the stethoscope bell onto Brooke's back and listened to each of the quadrants (sections) of her lungs as she inhaled and exhaled. High-pitched or windy noises when Brooke was breathing out meant her airways were obstructed. The doctor instructed me to note which quadrants were involved in the wheezing, as well as the pitch and loudness.

If I heard the squeaks or high-pitched sounds only at the end of expiration (breathing out), I knew that her attack was mild or just beginning. If I heard the high-pitched noises the whole time she breathed out, I knew that the attack was more serious.

I was to listen to Brooke, medicate her according to the doctor's instructions and then watch her for the next twenty

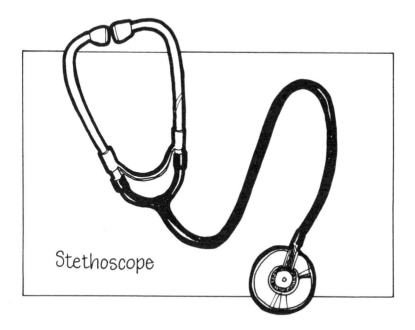

Stethoscope

to thirty minutes. If she did not improve, I had to take her to the doctor. If she did improve, I would continue the medications according to instructions.

Some young children are so accustomed to wheezing, they don't even know when they do it. In my experience, if your child is under three years old, the stethoscope will provide you with useful information for early intervention.

Once you have listened to your child's chest with the stethoscope, it will be important to report to your doctor the sounds you may have heard, as well as any of the following:

- Is your child's skin color normal?

- Check your child's lip color and fingernails. Gray or slightly blue coloring is a sign that your child is in great need of oxygen.

- Check the skin in the dip just above your child's collar-bone. Does it pull in as your child is breathing? This is a sign that your child is struggling to breathe.

- Check the rib cage and belly. If your little one is struggling to breathe, the muscles will pull in around the ribs and the belly will work harder to push the air out of the lungs.

If any of these signs is present and you heard wheezing when you used the stethoscope, you can be certain your child or baby needs medical attention *right away.*

I always take my stethoscope with us when Brooke goes to the pediatrician or to the hospital. I like to know what she sounds like before I take her home so I can compare it with the sound when we arrived.

By the way, if you intend to purchase a stethoscope, buy an inexpensive one. A simple nurse's stethoscope should cost between five and fifteen dollars. I paid twelve dollars for mine years ago and it still works fine.

Although a stethoscope is still very useful for parents of children over four years of age, at this age parents can begin using another tool which will provide an even earlier indication of breathing problems, a peak flow meter.

PEAK FLOW METERS

During an asthma attack or episode, the airways become narrow, restricting airflow. The peak flow meter, a hand-held instrument, was designed to measure the openness of the airways by gauging the airflow. Though many people have never heard of them, peak flow meters have been in use

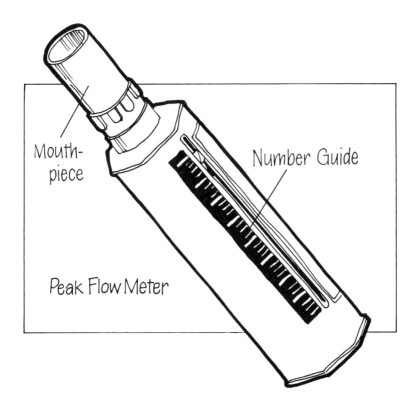

Mouth-
piece

Number Guide

Peak Flow Meter

(mostly in research settings) for roughly twenty years. The concept is much the same as that of any other medical instrument that provides objective information for patient evaluation.

In Chapter 4 I used the illustration which likened the usefulness of a peak flow meter to the usefulness of a thermometer to measure body temperature, a tire gauge to measure air pressure in a tire, and a gas gauge to measure the amount of gas in a car. Someday peak flow meters, too, will be common household items for people with asthma.

Peak flow meters are currently in use in hospitals, emergency rooms, doctors' offices, homes and schools. There are many practical uses for the peak flow meter in each setting. The peak flow meter can:

- confirm diagnosis of asthma

- confirm suspicions of exercise-induced asthma

- monitor patient's response to medication during an asthma flare

- monitor patient's response to asthma management plan

- provide objective information to parent for adjusting the asthma management plans according to doctor's instructions

- provide objective information to teachers and parents regarding sending the child to school and permissible activities

- provide the earliest indication of an approaching asthma attack or flare

- provide the parent with an opportunity to respond to an approaching attack with the least amount of interruption and intervention

- reinforce learning appropriate self-management skills for the child

- motivate children who, out of fear, may have avoided exercise altogether, to engage safely in normal exercise.

Believe it or not, this list could go on and on!

Flow meters are easy to use. The child simply takes a deep breath, puts her lips around the mouthpiece and blows as hard as she can. The force of her blow moves the spring-loaded indicator arrow along the metered shaft where it stops at the top of the expiration. This procedure is repeated two more times. The highest number achieved (not an average of the three blows) is then recorded. This number is then compared to the expected "normal" range.

The child's asthma management plan can be written by the doctor to correspond to the numbers on the peak flow meter. This system provides a common ground for communication between doctors and parents and patients as well as between the school, home and doctor's office. This system is relatively easy for a child to learn so that as he gets older he will be able to continue optimal management.

Don't be surprised if many of the doctors you run into do not yet know what a peak flow meter is. I became acquainted with flow meters when Brooke was part of the drug study program at Georgetown University Hospital. I had never heard of one before that time. I was so excited about what it taught me, I showed it to my pediatrician and now all the pediatricians in the office use peak flow meters for their asthma patients.

There are some doctors who are very reluctant to teach their patients to use a peak flow meter. These doctors are very knowledgeable regarding asthma management, but just do not understand the great freedom and psychological relief that peak flow meters provide to those of us who use them.

I travel around the country speaking to various groups, and it almost never fails that a parent will stand up and give testimony to the usefulness of the peak flow meter.

Not long ago, a group of us were busy folding, stapling and

stamping newsletters. Jane, a first-time volunteer, asked, "What do you do when your child is playing hard and you can tell he's beginning to have trouble and should use his inhaler, but he insists he's okay?" As if led by a conductor, Debbie (my assistant editor) and Janice (our faithful Girl Tuesday) said at once, "That's one reason to use a flow meter!"

They went on to discuss how letting the flow meter decide whether or not to medicate saves Mom or Dad from playing the heavy. The kid can't argue with the flow meter. Additionally, you can have him blow again about thirty minutes after he medicates and he'll be able to see by the improved reading on the flow meter how the medicine has opened up his airways. (Save this demonstration for another day if he's already out playing again!)

Flow meters can also help children who are afraid of having an asthma attack while exercising. Many of these children would rather avoid the exercise than to be embarrassed by an attack in front of friends. If the peak flow meter reading is normal and no wheezing is present, gentle encouragement to take prescribed medication according to the doctor's instruction *before* exercising and then participate (even if at a low level) will open up doors of freedom for children who live in fear of impending attacks. Building lung capacity, important for asthmatics, is difficult if there is fear that exercise will induce an attack.

There are many wonderful examples of how people are successfully using peak flow meters to implement their asthma management plans. But even though peak flow meters have been in use for almost twenty years, there is only one book written specifically for doctors on the subject. This book, which can be understood by parents or adult patients, is called *Peak Performance* and was written by Guillermo

Mendoza, M.D., this country's leading expert in peak flow monitoring. (Dr. Mendoza also co-authored with Debbie Scherrer and me a handbook on peak flow monitoring for the consumer entitled, *A User's Guide to Peak Flow Monitoring.* If you are interested in obtaining copies of either of these books, they are available through Mothers of Asthmatics. See the Resource section.)

Debbie Scherrer, who learned right from the source about peak flow meters, recently related this story:

> *"For years my children's asthma kept us awake and frightened night after night, only to 'disappear' by the time we would see the doctor the next day. It had been a great frustration to me. Finally, at a patient education workshop sponsored by the Asthma and Allergy Foundation of America, the presentation by Dr. Guillermo Mendoza of Los Angeles clarified the problem and its solution. It was like music to my ears.*
>
> *"He was talking about asthma symptoms, which worsen at night. Studies have shown that lung function has a cyclical nature. It follows a pattern that when charted looks like a curve that peaks in the afternoon and dips to its lowest point between midnight and 6 A.M. The reason for this pattern is not totally clear, but part of the explanation includes the fact that during these hours the body's production of its own cortisone and adrenaline is 'in low gear,' and the body's prone position allows for the accumulation of mucus in the airways.*
>
> *"He went on to say that lots of kids look great during the day, yet night after night they have serious problems. A typical scenario is this—a mom spends a frantic night dealing with her child's asthma. She medicates,*

hydrates, props, rocks, and worries, and they manage to make it through the night. By the time they see the doctor during regular office hours, the child has reached the high point of his lung function curve. The doctor, using a stethoscope for his examination, pronounces the child to be fine, suspects the mom of being a kook and sends them home to face another frightening night. The irony, Dr. Mendoza stated, is that the next time, the mother's frustration might even cause her to withhold the child's morning dose of medication in the hope that the child will wheeze for the doctor and convince him that there really is a problem.

"I couldn't believe it! He was describing my children's early asthma experiences as accurately as if he had been there! I've never told anyone, but I had even resorted to the 'medicine game' myself to try to avoid strange looks from the doctor. Not only did I begin to question my own judgment after several of these 'perfectly fine' office visits, but my children were deprived of the full-time medication schedule they needed to bring their asthma under control. At the time I thought I was surely the only one in the world living that kind of nightmare, but from the number of heads bobbing around the room as Dr. Mendoza spoke, I could see that I had not been alone.

"All the frustration could have been avoided with one simple device—a peak flow meter. If the doctor had used one along with his stethoscope in his office evaluations, he would have been able to tell that my 'perfectly fine' child was operating at about only 80 percent of his breathing capacity. (A stethoscope will only detect a problem with a drop of approximately 25 percent or more.) If he had taught me how to use one at home I

would have been able to report to him how things progressed at night—that at 11 P.M. the child would wake up coughing and choking with a peak flow reading of ____, which would improve to ____ after medication, then would bottom out around 3 A.M. at ____, after which the child would settle down and sleep until morning. The peak flow measurements could have been easily charted for the doctor to interpret and design a treatment plan that would have quickly put an end to all those sleepless nights. Sounds simple, and it is.

"I wish it had been that easy for me and my children. We lived the nightmare far too long, until change to a new doctor, asthma education, a peak flow meter and the proper treatment plan brought their asthma under control. If you are presently in an out-of-control situation, Dr. Mendoza's message should be music to your ears, too. In terms of the frustration and medical expenses you are experiencing, a peak flow meter is a cheap investment you will be glad to make. If you're worried that it might be too 'high tech' for you to master, forget it! If your child is at least four years old he can blow into it, and the result is easier to read than a thermometer. The key is to work with a doctor who is up to date on the most recent advances in asthma treatment and is willing to teach you the proper use of the medications and techniques that will bring you the freedom of control. Don't settle for less!

"Dr. Mendoza also emphasized that once control is achieved, the flow meter is a valuable tool in helping the doctor to reduce the amount of medications needed to maintain optimum lung function. As medications are tapered, the parent monitors the child regularly and is prepared to reinstate higher dosing levels at the first

sign of a drop. This eliminates the reservations that plague all parents who are naturally reluctant to continue 'pumping in' unnecessary medications."

Most companies manufacture a low flow range peak flow meter for children and a full range meter for adults. For children under five years of age, a low range flow meter is fine, but if your child is above age five, a durable full range peak flow will be a worthwhile investment.

A quality flow meter should be constructed of durable material that resists breakage when dropped (because it *will* get dropped and some peak flow meters break easily), be easily transportable, have a definitive measurement scale and should be made by a company with a reputation for reliability. Check warranties, too. A good product should last several years. We have had ours for four years and it still works great.

There is a flow meter available which some children as young as two years old have been able to use that has a whistle to motivate the child to blow as hard as he can. Dr. Thomas Plaut, author of the recently revised *Children with Asthma: A Manual for Parents,* tested this flow meter, the Peak Flow Monitor, in his practice and told me that to everyone's delight he had a thirty-two-month-old child using it effectively.

The stethoscope and peak flow meter are both useful in *monitoring* your child's health. Now we will examine nebulizer compressors and spacers, tools of the trade that assist in the *delivery* of medication.

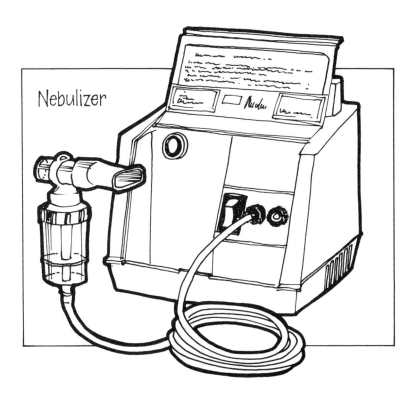

Nebulizer

NEBULIZERS

Nebulizer compressors, commonly called breathing machines, are portable air compressors that transform a liquid medication into a mist. The mist is then inhaled by the patient. Medicines typically used in nebulizer compressors are Alupent (metaproterenol), Brethaire (terbutaline), Bronkosol (isoetharine), Intal (cromolyn sodium), Proventil and Ventolin (albuterol), and Atrovent (ipratropium bromide).

If your child has ever been hospitalized or required emergency room service, you are probably familiar with breathing treatments. Home use of the nebulizer can actually reduce the number of unscheduled doctor's office visits and emergency room situations and admissions.

Generally speaking, nebulizer compressors are wonderful because they put the medication where it is needed. If your child fell and scraped his knee, you wouldn't spray disinfectant over his entire body. Certain medicines are most effective when applied topically (on the lungs in this case) rather than ingested.

Some, *but not all*, medications used with the nebulizer compressor have mild side effects. Make sure you understand dosing and frequency of treatments each time you receive instructions from your doctor.

Asthma medications are potent medications. Underuse *or* overuse (not following doctor's orders) can put your child in serious danger. I consider the opportunity to have a nebulizer compressor at home an honor. It is a privilege I earned.

HOW A NEBULIZER WORKS

The motor pump filters air through the machine and into clear plastic tubing that leads to a medicine cup called a nebulizer cup. The liquid medicine is placed into the cup and the cap is placed on top. The mask or mouthpiece which directs the medication to the face attaches to the opening in the top of the nebulizer cup and the machine is turned on. The patient places the mask over the nose and mouth. The patient then breathes slowly and deeply until the misting stops, indicating that the medication has been delivered. The length of delivery varies from one unit to another but most nebulizer treatments take about seven to ten minutes.

Brooke not only needs to have a nebulizer compressor at home, but her doctor believes I am capable of using it properly. If your doctor prescribes a nebulizer compressor, be responsible!

Several types of nebulizer compressors are available, and new models seem to be developed by the manufacturers almost every year. The standard nebulizer consists of a motor with a filter, masking, and tubing and uses standard household electrical current. Other models offer such options as a nasal tip to direct the medication into the nasal passages, the option to take a treatment while lying down and adapters for plugging into a car cigarette lighter. Some models operate on a self-contained battery. Some units are bulkier than others. Some are disguised to look like a lunch pail or are carried in a lightweight shoulder bag while others look very institutional.

If your child is preschool age or younger, a home nebulizer compressor which offers the luxury of letting him recline while taking the breathing treatment will be a great asset. If your child plays little league sports, is involved in camping or other outdoor activity, the freedom a portable battery-operated unit will provide him will be worth the extra cost. But sometimes it is difficult to find a unit that does all things and does them well. It may even be necessary to purchase two nebulizer compressors to meet the needs of your child.

A Word of Caution: There is a sonic nebulizer machine which uses ultrasound to break up the particles of medicine to be inhaled as a mist. It is a quiet unit, but as the manufacturer suggests, it should not be used by asthma patients because in some patients the particles produced by the machine can actually induce an asthma attack.

Regardless of looks or fancy options, a nebulizer is one piece of equipment which should come with a hefty warranty. The two major companies I deal with (see Resources section) are proud of their reputation to replace nebulizer compressors that fail to live up to the customer's expectations. Those companies that believe in their product are also willing to stand behind it. Buy quality first, options second. The warranty is important because this will be a big purchase. Nebulizer compressors cost anywhere from $125 to $350.

Use the Resources section of this book to write to the various manufacturers for information. When making a purchase of this magnitude, follow your doctor's recommendation or shop around and base your decision on quality (check the warranty), options and cost. If it looks as if you will need two nebulizer compressors, purchase the one that meets most of your needs first and later buy the one with the options you can live without for a while. Nebulizer compressors, when prescribed by a doctor, are tax deductible along with your other medical expenses unless you are reimbursed by your health insurance for the cost.

Some insurance companies cover the purchase price of a nebulizer compressor but most do not. I believe this is a sad mistake. If more health insurance companies would recognize the nebulizer's great potential for reducing emergency room visits, hospitalizations and unscheduled sick visits to the doctor, their enormous asthma-related financial liability would be greatly reduced.

Purchase replacement nebulizer cups and additional tubing and filters when ordering your nebulizer compressor. There are about a dozen different models of nebulizer cups— Puritan Bennett, Hospitak, Marquest, Diverse Pulmonary and Mountain Medical, to name just a few of them. Assembly packets can be customized to include a mouthpiece instead of a mask or vice versa. Most assembly packets contain everything you need, but one nice feature you should check on is a thumb port or a tee piece that allows you to use intermittent inhaled therapy. The thumb port allows the child to control the flow of medication and reduces waste. Assembly packets can be purchased through allergy supply companies as well.

It is important to keep the machine clean, to replace the masking, nebulizer cup and tubing often and to keep medications sterile. Contaminants that get into medications or saline solution (used to dilute medications) or that remain in overused tubing are inhaled by the patient along with the medications.

After each breathing treatment, rinse the disassembled nebulizer cup and mask in warm running water for about thirty seconds. Shake the mask and cup parts to remove large droplets of water and allow them to air dry on a clean towel (or paper towel). Once dry, put the nebulizer cup and mask in a Ziploc bag and store it in a safe, accessible place. (We store ours in a small rectangular basket in the kitchen cabinet above the sink.) Roll up the tubing and store it inside the nebulizer case if a space is provided. Otherwise, put it in a Ziploc bag and store it next to the mask and nebulizer cup. Tubing should be replaced often because it is hard to clean and harbors moisture. If the tubing becomes cloudy, you've used it too long. Replacement cups, masking and tubing are available from medical supply companies and the manufacturers of nebulizer compressors.

If your child uses the nebulizer compressor daily, use the following cleaning procedure every other day. Otherwise, follow these directions every *six to eight treatments:* Wash the disassembled nebulizer cup and mask with a mild dish soap and warm water. Rinse all the parts well using warm, running tap water. Mix together one cup of vinegar and two cups of water. Soak the nebulizer parts in the solution for thirty minutes. Rinse in warm water for one minute, shake off water droplets, let air dry and store in a Ziploc bag.

INHALERS

A metered-dose inhaler is a canister of medicine which ejects a medicated mist into the patient's airways. Ask your doctor to teach your child the correct way to use the inhaler. He will show your child how to stand up straight, take a deep breath, blow all his air out, put the inhaler in front of his mouth, depress the inhaler canister and immediately inhale slowly and deeply. If you notice medicine getting sprayed around your child's face, don't assume that enough medication has gone into his lungs.

Keep the inhaler clean and free of medication buildup by rinsing it daily and washing it with mild detergent weekly. Always keep the cap on when not in use.

For children or arthritic adults who have trouble working the metered-dose inhaler and inhaling the medication at the same time, Allen and Hanburys division of Glaxo has a handy gadget called the VentEase. The VentEase is a squeeze trigger which fits over the plastic sleeve of Ventolin and Beclovent inhalers. Children like them because they really do make using an inhaler easier. The VentEase is also a handy stand for the inhaler.

SPACERS

A spacer extends the space between a metered-dose inhaler and the mouth of the patient. It is a chamber which traps the particles of medication long enough for the patient to inhale two or three times. Several studies have shown that the use of a spacer improves the delivery of the medication to the lungs and therefore improves its effectiveness.

Doctors often prescribe the use of a spacer for patients who have trouble coordinating the aim of the metered-dose inhaler, depressing the canister and inhaling the product. If the medication is deposited on the back of the throat or on the tongue, enough of the medicine will not reach the lungs and it won't work properly.

There are several different spacer models available but all of them basically do the same thing. I prefer a model that is easy to carry, is inexpensive and easy to master. Some children who use flow meters have problems remembering to inhale instead of exhale if they use a spacer similar in shape to a flow meter. Some spacers can be taken apart for cleaning while others must be thrown away after they've been used awhile. A few patients using inhaled steroids sometimes develop hoarseness, thrush (also called candidiasis) in the mouth and throat. This is thought to be caused by the medication being improperly deposited on the tongue or back of the throat. Many patients are relieved of this problem when they use a spacer.

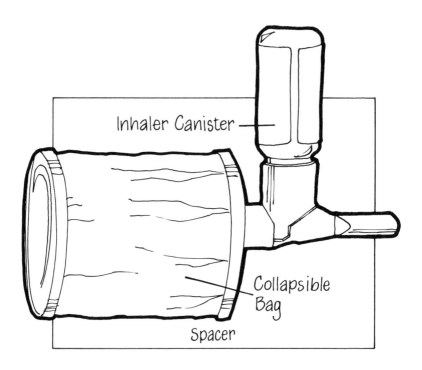

Inhaler Canister

Collapsible Bag

Spacer

OTHER TOOLS

If your child is having trouble breathing and you suspect a fever, don't torture the kid with a mercury thermometer. Try a digital battery-operated one. You can buy one for about $6.00 at a drugstore.

Water Pik by Teledyne can be adapted for use as a nasal irrigator and is very effective in treating allergy patients who have chronic sinusitis. It requires a special nasal attachment and sterile saline solution. Our otolaryngologist (ear, nose and throat doctor) prescribed it for Brooke when she was six years old to combat chronic sinus infections which were triggering her asthma. She had been on a constant dose of antibiotics and antihistamines and required office treatments for her sinuses until she started using the Water Pik as a nasal irrigator.

The procedure may cause minor discomfort in the form of pressure for a moment even if done correctly. However, minor discomfort for the moment can help reduce your child's dependence on medications to control asthma. If your doctor prescribes this type of treatment, follow the instructions for keeping all parts of the machine sterile. Water Pik can be purchased at most variety or department stores. The nasal attachment must be ordered through your (OTO) doctor.

There are other methods of nasal irrigation which your doctor may suggest. Generally speaking, however, nasal irrigation is not a daily event.

In addition to these tools, there are germicides, cold air masks (great for joggers during winter months or for children who want to play in the snow), hygrometers to measure indoor humidity levels and barometers (for weather-sensitive asthmatics). There are also lots of products that claim to reduce allergens in the environment. You'll learn about many of these in the next chapter.

CHAPTER 7

ALLERGY-PROOFING
YOUR HOME

ALLERGEN AVOIDANCE IS VITAL TO GAIN CONTROL over allergic asthma. It does no good to feed your child a multitude of medications while overlooking this step. Recently, I saw a news film about a child who had asthma and allergies and great difficulty in coping with them. She missed a lot of school and the parents were trying to get the school system to provide a homebound tutor for her. However, the child's bedroom was one huge allergy pit. It was cluttered with papers and clothes and generally unkempt. On the table was an enormous supply of pills and equipment. As much as I could sympathize with the child, a barrelful of asthma medications, air filters, nebulizer compressors and flow meters will not control asthma which is continually aggravated by accumulating allergens. Nor should the child's school be expected to provide home tutoring for the child when the parents are unwilling to provide a healthful home environment for her to live (and learn) in.

But I don't recommend, as many instruction sheets do, that you seal off your child's bedroom closet with plastic sheeting or that your child should be subjected to a room in which he cannot express his personality either. Just clean, uncluttered and maintained. The more clutter that is in the way, the more difficult it is to clean.

Often the subject of environmental controls evokes feelings of frustration because changing one's living habits is initially very difficult. Together we will address each stage of allergen control, and if you begin to feel a bit overwhelmed, put the book down and repeat these words slowly three times: All I can be expected to do is the best that I am able right now. Then pick the book back up and continue reading. No white tornado is going to knock at your door. You don't have to call a contractor to rebuild your home and your life. Just take one step at a time.

TACKLING THE BEDROOM

Your child spends between eight and fourteen out of every twenty-four hours in her bedroom. At least eight of those hours are spent sleeping with what could be one of the cul-

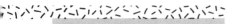

prits of her asthma, *dust mites*. Dust mites are microscopic creatures that feast on flakes of our dead skin while we sleep soundly in our beds. Everyone has them in their beds, even the President of the United States.

Pillow and mattress encasings make it easier to avoid dust mites. The encasings protect the child from the dust mites living on the mattress and pillow. Most people are unaffected by dust mites but to those who are allergic to them, the encasings are a great blessing.

Until recently, you could only purchase crinkly vinyl-lined encasings to protect mattresses and pillows from dust mites. You were supposed to fit a bed sheet and pillow case over the liners and tell your child to have sweet dreams. They were hot in the summer and cold in the winter and sounded very uncozy when you tucked your slumber bug into bed. Also, the vinyl was prone to tears, so before long, holes larger than mites started appearing.

Now there are vinyl fabrics that are more flexible and some that are cotton polyester on one side and vinyl on the other. We really like our mattress and pillow encasings because they look like, feel like and wash like what people like to sleep on.

We encased Brooke's box springs as well. Check the Resources section of this book for purchasing information. If the doctor has prescribed mattress and pillow encasings, they are a tax deductible medical expense. Besides using encasings, wash all bedding in very hot water weekly to make sure you kill the mites.

huge stuffed toys to take home,
Without mother insisting while the children groan.
When you met me, you'd notice I smell of perfume
And not vinegar water, which now scents the rooms.
Now please understand that I do love the kids
With their wheezes and noses and pharmacy bills

But I dream, oh, I dream what would our life be
If I never had heard of the word "allergy."

—Betsy Koch, Newsletter Editor, The Allentown Asthma and Allergy Support Group, Allentown, Pennsylvania

If your child must share the room with another child, both children must have few or no toys tucked on shelves or under beds. Both beds will need encasings and pets should be kept out of the room. A room air filter may help, especially if there is no "whole house" filter. Replace heavy drapes and venetian blinds with lightweight washable curtains and remember to wash them regularly. Or use shades. Furniture should be kept to a minimum and the tops should be kept clear and wiped with a damp or oiled cloth at least once a week. Vacuum the whole house and especially the bedroom regularly, preferably while the child is not home. Keep pictures, even those that are framed and washable, to a minimum. Windows at least in the bedroom (but preferably in the whole house) should be kept closed at all times during the offending pollen season. Above all, do not smoke in the house, and especially not in your child's room.

Changes to the bedroom will be accepted better if they are made while our children are too young to know the difference, but if you are making changes that mean beloved Teddy must sleep in another room (stuffed animals harbor all kinds of allergens, including dust mites), then tread carefully. I made the mistake of telling five-year-old Brooke we would need to put her smaller stuffed animals (gifts from well-meaning friends) in Ziploc bags when she was not playing with them. What I thought was such a logical, wonderful idea caused a sudden flood of tears! "I'd rather give them away than put them where they won't be able to breathe," she sobbed.

Instead, we found a plastic toy box with a lid and put them in there until, as even little children do, she forgot about them and they gradually found a new home. (Don't anyone tell Brooke, please!) To detract from my major goof-up, we ordered some pretty pink heart wallpaper with a teddy bear border. Her knickknacks are housed in a glass-enclosed lawyer's bookshelf. Forbidden treasures still have a mysterious way of finding Brooke's room, so periodically I have to pay a visit and haul them all away. Don't most moms? It is a fine balance we must strike in our efforts to keep their rooms as allergy-free as possible without wiping out their developing personalities.

AIR FILTERS

Selecting the right air filter can be totally overwhelming. There are so many models, each with its particular features and efficiency ratings. Every company claims that its product is the best but how do you know which one is right for your situation?

It helps to remember that there are three basic types of filters. One is a HEPA (High Efficiency Particulate Actuation) filter, a nonelectric unit which cleans the air as it passes through several special filters. It is very efficient at removing most particles floating in the air, but it cannot filter out gases or bacteria. Most HEPA units are portable.

Electrostatic filters charge or electrocute the particles as they pass into the filter. The particles are then trapped in the aluminum mesh filter which can be removed and cleaned every few weeks. These units can fit into the existing filter slot in your heating system, or they can be professionally installed in the ductwork of your house. They filter bacteria and viruses as well as smoke, odors and gaseous fumes (ours turned itself on when we painted our basement floor!). The only drawback is that this unit emits ozone, which can be a problem for a minority of kids with asthma. Check the literature or ask the sales representative about this.

The third type of filter is the common fiberglass disposable filter that you change every few weeks. The trouble with fiberglass is that microscopic particles of the filter also make their way into the air that we breathe. Also, they allow many particles of dust and other allergens to recirculate. This is the least appropriate filter for children with asthma.

Within these three categories, there are models that are portable, console, whole house and room size. The best way to decide which filter is best for your situation is to ask your doctor for a recommendation. Call a local rental store or allergy supply company and see if they have a portable unit you can rent for a month. Keep the air filter running constantly. See how much "stuff" it filters, and if there is a noticeable improvement in your child's asthma. Check furniture surfaces to see if less dust settles. Some filter companies have a rental plan with an option to buy their filter included in the agreement.

If it becomes evident that an air filter is necessary, try to determine which kind of filter will be best suited for your child and still fit into your heating system. In our case, we purchased an electrostatic air filter through the catalogue department at Montgomery Ward in 1982 and have had very good results. We also have a portable HEPA unit for Brooke's room for extra benefit.

In making your purchase consider, as we did, the filter efficiency ratings, which are determined in part by the filter's ability to remove the most minute particles of pollen and bacteria. These particles are measured in microns, a unit of measure equal to one millionth of a meter. Ninety-nine percent of airborne particles are smaller than one micron. Most ordinary air filters remove only those particles that are ten microns or larger.

If you are renting the home or apartment you live in, you may want to purchase a portable unit or one that simply replaces the furnace filter and then take it with you when you move (but beware: filter sizes vary among furnaces).

If you install a whole-house unit in your heating and cooling system, be sure to mention this fact to your realtor when you sell your home. Options such as these don't necessarily raise the value of your home but may make it more attractive to potential buyers.

Discuss the matter of purchasing a filter with your child's allergist or pediatrician, as it is usually a major expense. Units that plug into your heating/cooling system cost from just under one hundred dollars to six hundred dollars depending on the accessibility and age of your system and on how many options the filtering units have. Portable units are usually the same amount or less. Shop around, and ask whether your doctor can purchase them any less expensively than you can. Don't settle for the little plastic tabletop drugstore variety of air filter. Buy quality at an affordable price, and check the warranty. Do not buy unless there is a money-back guarantee in writing. Also, the cost of certain filters that meet specific standards are tax deductible or may be reimbursed by health insurance.

A general rule of thumb in purchasing filter units is: if the pollution is coming from outside (pollen, etc.), a central filter is best. If it is coming from inside (a smoking parent), the room unit may be best.

Whatever your situation, an air filter is not a replacement for taking other steps to reduce allergens in the air. Your child's room must still be kept free of clutter, and be dusted and vacuumed frequently, and the sheets should be changed weekly. Filters must be changed or cleaned frequently. Family pets must still be kept out of the child's bedroom and it's very important to have your home air ducts cleaned every two to three years, more often if you live in dusty, humid, pollen-ridden areas of the country. Newly constructed homes should have their ductwork cleaned right away to remove construction debris, dry wall dust and, sometimes, lunch trash left by workmen.

After I was on the "Today" show, I received a call from Craig Hitchcock, president of the National Institute of Furnace and Air Duct Cleaning Specialists. He offered his assistance in helping *MA Report* readers understand the importance of clean air in their homes. He sent us several photographs which we published with descriptive captions. One was of a box of debris that was left in the air ducts by builders of one home for over three years prior to cleaning the ductwork. The estimated weight? Twenty-eight pounds!

What you can't see can hurt you! Few of us ever look into our heating and cooling ducts with flashlights to see what grunge grows there. If you think mold and mildew confine themselves to damp basements, guess again. Every once in a while, we get letters from parents who swear there is some invisible trigger floating in the air of their home or school that is causing their child's asthma symptoms. The truth is, they could be right.

It is a mistake to think that our heating and cooling systems push air through sleek shiny columns or tubes of sheet metal. Contaminants most often found in home heating and cooling systems are aspergillus (brownish-gray) and penicillium molds (white), both of which can be allergens for some people.

Gas and oil are less clean fuels than electric heat. "In fact," says Mr. Hitchcock, "gas is especially dirty. Gas is a cooler-burning heat so it develops condensation which causes the furnace to rust. Rust furthers corrosion as it builds up in the furnace. This can cause cracks and other damage resulting in a carbon monoxide buildup in your home. Since the gas is colorless and odorless, it may not be detected until it is too late."

Mr. Hitchcock cited an example that occurred in 1986 when a doctor and his five children died in their sleep after a faulty furnace leaked the gas throughout their home. Some people are sensitive to gas fumes and detect them whereas others, unaware of the fumes, may experience symptoms that are often incorrectly diagnosed.

One woman went to the doctor to be tested for allergies. She tested negative. When the ductwork and furnace were cleaned, the workmen found a four-and-a-half-inch crack in the heat exchanger, which caused carbon monoxide to be pulled into the ductwork throughout the house. When the problem with the furnace was fixed, so were her "allergies." Lingering flu symptoms also often plague people who have contaminated air ducts.

Homeowners should check air ducts with a flashlight. Simply remove the vent covers and look inside. If you don't see molds or dust accumulating there, check beyond where the filter goes in (the box called the plenum). If you don't see anything there, so far so good. Take off the heat vents on your floor, walls and ceiling and check in there. If you already have an air-filtering system installed and you notice that there is still a large buildup of dust on the furniture between dustings, this is a good sign that it is time for you to wash or change your filters or have your system checked or cleaned. The cost of cleaning varies according to region, *so be sure to check prices before you schedule the work.* Mr. Hitchcock said a good average estimate could be based on between ten to thirteen dollars per duct and clean air returns. This fee includes cleaning the system as well as the ductwork. A good air duct cleaning company will be equipped with a big vacuum truck and will use high-compressed air as well.

Clean air ducts improve fuel efficiency, as well as provide a more allergen-free environment. A healthy heating and cooling system ensures against other hazards such as poisonous-fume leaks. Though the service may seem expensive, it is, when contrasted with the high cost of disease, worth it!

Though this is not to be taken as an endorsement of this company, you may obtain more information regarding this service by writing or calling Mr. Hitchcock at his Oklahoma office: Mr. Craig Hitchcock, Southwest Power Vac, P.O. Box 811, Norman, OK 73070; 405-321-0289.

VACUUMS

Don't you wish we could vacuum the allergies away? Maybe we can't get rid of all the allergens but we can suck a few of them into a dust bag and toss them away. We can, that is, with the help of a vacuum cleaner specially designed to meet standards that your nose will notice. These are called allergy vacuums.

While the concept of an allergy vacuum is fantastic, they usually are far more expensive than the average department store variety. Therefore, the Mothers of Asthmatics staff researched and tested three out of five portable allergy vacuums. The two vacuums we eliminated required elaborate, messy and time-consuming measures to maintain and the cost of the units was higher than the three models we selected to test. So which three models did we test? The Miele 234i, Nilfisk GS90 and the Vita-Vac. We put these machines to the test in the homes of people who have real live allergies.

First we tried the Vita-Vac, made by the Vita-Mix Corporation. From the outside, the tank looks like a souped-up Electrolux. When you open the tank to look inside you see quite a different story. It has a triple-walled bag to catch the dust and a unique HEPA filtering system to catch anything that may escape the bag. Each time we changed a bag, we wiped our hands along the inside of the canister and it was still as clean as the day it arrived. Even after one of the testers used it to vacuum the leftover ashes out of her fireplace! (We don't recommend using any vacuum for this purpose on a regular basis, though.)

Another feature about the dust bag we liked was its system for disposal. The Vita-Vac dust bags come with an adhesive disk. Peel off one side of the disk, smack it over the hole at the top of the bag (before removing it from the canister) and lift the bag out of the vacuum without ever getting your hands dirty. And I bet you can't do this with your vacuum . . . run the vacuum engine with the canister and dust bag open. Do this with the Vita-Vac and the dust stays put.

I think that all of us who tried the Vita-Vac liked the dust collection and disposal properties of the vacuum best. There is nothing fancy about the attachments and it is easy to transport and store. It is also easy to vacuum stairs. The directions say you should only need to change the bag six times a year. Either we all have very dirty houses or someone needs to double that number.

Though the Vita-Vac does a great job of picking up the dust and dirt, it might be nice to have a few other features such as variable speeds for vacuuming drapes, a retractable cord or a storage caddy for attachments. But the vacuum is very nice and will do a good job for you.

Next, we tested the Miele (Mee-lay), which happens to be the least expensive of the three. Fresh out of the box, it looked mighty fancy. It is lightweight, the attachments are first-class and it is relatively quiet. Upon opening the canister, we found the dust-filtering bag and two other filters. This vacuum does have some nice features that the other two did not. It has a nifty attachment for cleaning drapes, between blinds and under hard to reach places (like the piano). All the attachments are stored within the canister. The telescoping metal wand can be adjusted to the height of the user. The attachments stay securely in place once attached to the vacuum. There is a "bag is full, you dummy" indicator on the machine.

While on the subject of the bag indicator, the vacuum hose became clogged several times during testing, but the only way we could tell was that the bag-is-full indicator showed red for no apparent reason. The bag was not full and the suction seemed absolutely fine. We were only able to determine that the hose was indeed actually clogged by dropping a marble or penny into it and note where it stopped. The three times it did clog, it happened in the handle portion only and was very easily remedied.

We did not like the fact that the exhaust air on the Miele blew upward into your face if you walked behind the machine. And while we are sure that the filtering system is allergy adequate, it does not rival that of the Vita-Vac. I also disliked changing the bag and filters because my hands could and did get dirty. I used a mailing label sticker to cover the hole of the dust bag to keep the dirt inside but the other two filters got pretty dirty between changes. Several of our testers noted that the process of changing attachments was cumbersome and time consuming. One tester claimed the "telescoping wand" nearly drove her to distraction, and she finally gave up trying to change its length.

Just about the time I was through testing the Miele and ready to pass it on to the next tester, I plugged in my Hoover canister to clean up a rather dusty, dirty mess. (I didn't want to use the good one for it.) I no sooner plugged it in than I was convinced that allergy vacs really *do* make a difference! My eyes, nose and lungs could tell the difference and I don't have asthma or allergies. The other testers made similar discoveries as well.

Last to arrive was the Nilfisk. It is lightweight, has some very nice attachments, is sturdy, easy to assemble and does a very quiet, nice job of sucking up what it's supposed to. We ordered one with a HEPA filter, an optional feature for added filtering, which we had to install ourselves. (No sweat!) This filter must be replaced once every five years. There is no retractable cord but we really didn't mind because it is a heavy-duty rubber-coated cord, one which did not give us a problem with tangling.

The canister is made of lightweight, high-impact plastic and glided easily over any surfaces in our homes. One nice feature each of us enjoyed was the fact that it didn't send exhaust air blowing around the room. However, the regular dust bag is big and awkward to change.

We liked Nilfisk's air-activated beater-bar attachment for rugs. There were no extra cords to change or attach and it did an excellent job. We liked the floor-nozzle attachment, which, like the Miele, let you go from hard surface floors to rugs (short pile) with but a slight touch of your toe. The attachments are stored in a holder you can hang on the wall in your utility room or closet.

So which did we like the best? There were features about each that we loved and, if the truth be known, we'd be happy with any one of them. The important lesson we each learned is that these vacuums are serious machines and deliver a quality clean.

Having been a skeptic before embarking upon this research project, I am fully convinced that I will never use a vacuum in my home again unless it is an "allergy vacuum." You can almost taste the difference.

Now, if you are interested in a more scientific study of this great vacuum dilemma, write Mike McGrath, editor of *Allergy Relief*. Send $1.00 for his special report on allergy vacuums, which lists prices as well as technical information that will be helpful in making your decision on which vacuum to buy. Write: *Rodale's Allergy Relief*, 33 East Minor Street, Emmaus, PA 18049.

While not necessarily considered an allergy vacuum, *central vacuum systems* are often recommended by doctors because they deposit dust and exhaust in a canister located in a garage or basement instead of filtering the air in a tank that you pull along with you. Central vacuum systems are built behind the walls or in ductwork. Tubing runs from the motor throughout the house with wall outlets in several locations. The motor is activated when you plug the vacuum hose into the outlet and turn on a switch.

Some people say central vacuum systems aren't as powerful as portable units but after doing some sleuthing I found that, as usual, results depend on the quality of the system (not necessarily how much it costs). For homes with thick carpets, it may be necessary to purchase a model that has a motorized floor nozzle. With some models it is necessary to empty the collection tank frequently to ensure maximum power from the motor.

There are studies that indicate the central vacuum may indeed be less likely to stir up the dust while in use than a regular canister or upright vacuum. We considered having a central vacuum installed several years ago. If we had it installed while our house was being built, it would have cost about the same as any other quality vacuum. Having it installed later increases the price drastically. Check the Yellow Pages in your area and shop around for quality and price.

If the price of an allergy vacuum is more than your budget can handle right now, a good interim product may be a specially designed filter for your current vacuum. There is a product called Vacu-Filt, a filtering material which is like that found in allergy vacuum filters. Check the Resources section of this book for the product company you can order from.

STOP SMOKING

If you are a smoking parent of a child with asthma or allergies—*stop smoking! You are hurting your child.*

All across the country people are smacking this book shut and crying out in agony, "Why is she doing this to me?" Yes, they liked this book until now but they are saying things like, "I don't want to hear this again. Is there no place of refuge? I can't quit smoking. I've tried and I can't do it. Besides it is my body . . ." And then, they will rationalize the calming effect of the cigarette as they light up.

You *can stop smoking!* Smoking is an addictive behavior, according to the Surgeon General. We've been sold a product through advertising for years that hooks us and our families into a miserable, expensive, dangerous habit.

As hard as it may seem, it is possible to stop smoking— even though many people develop what Dr. Bob Lanier calls a "circular logic pattern." "I can't stop smoking because I'll gain weight, I can't gain weight, therefore I can't stop smoking." Another pattern: "Smoking calms my nerves. A cigarette is a friend who comforts me when I'm down and celebrates with me during the good times." Does that smack of a dependent attitude?

New techniques have been developed using chewing gums that help smokers wean themselves from cigarettes. If you've tried Nicorette and failed, chances are you were not properly instructed. Try again, but insist that the doctor teach you its proper use.

Medications used for lowering blood pressure have recently been found to dramatically reduce the craving suffered by many smokers. This medicine (a potent prescription item) is called "Catapress" and is administered through a skin patch. Discuss it with your doctor as a means of lessening withdrawal symptoms. Since the period of withdrawal is so severe for many people, many doctors feel that if there ever was a legitimate place for the short-term use of minor tranquilizers, the withdrawal period is it!

Some people do it cold turkey, some use hypnosis. Some have even been successful with acupuncture. If you are serious about your child's asthma, you will find a way to stop smoking. Ask your doctor and find a support group like the American Cancer Society for help. Just do it!!

What's the big deal about what smoking does to your child? A lung transfers oxygen from inhaled air to the bloodstream and exhales the waste product, carbon dioxide. The lungs of people who have asthma have difficulty supplying the blood with enough oxygen because some of the air is trapped in the outer areas of the lung where the transfer takes place, thus not leaving room to allow the fresh air in.

When there is carbon monoxide (a by-product of cigarette smoking) in the air taken in, it competes with oxygen to reach the red blood cells. Because of its chemical nature, carbon monoxide attaches itself to red blood cells about a hundred times more easily than oxygen, preventing the available oxygen from getting into the blood. Our children have enough trouble oxygenating their blood without the added burden of cigarette smoke.

Another problem with cigarette smoke is that it acts as an irritant to the lungs. In this capacity, smoke can trigger asthma through the same mechanism by which fumes and other irritants trigger asthma attacks.

Picture your three-year-old with a cigarette hanging out of her mouth. Pretty ridiculous, isn't it? It's just as ridiculous for you to expect her to live in a home where one or more adults pollute the air. Children are subject to the surroundings in which they are raised. They do not have the option of standing outside while you smoke. They do not have the option of avoiding the ashes and remnants of cigarettes scattered in trays about the house.

If I sound hard, it's because I constantly encounter parents who keep right on smoking despite all the evidence. Nothing is more frustrating than to help a family obtain a peak flow meter or nebulizer compressor when the family cannot afford to do it on its own, only to find out that the parents can afford the cigarettes that keep their child fighting for his breath. Parents share their stories of not being able to work because their child is always sick and yet some of them covet their right to smoke more than their child's health.

Then there are doctors who say, "Don't tell parents not to smoke because they won't give it up. Tell them to smoke outside . . ." It is a start but I do not know many people who continue to smoke outside of the house and never, ever inside. If this is the best effort parents can muster for their child, then it is certainly better than nothing at all. However, you should take steps to rid your house of any remnants of smoke odor. Strip the house of drapes, curtains, bedspreads, clothing in storage and drawers and have them cleaned or wash them completely. Then, using a cleaning solution that does not have strong vapors (no ammonia or chlorine and *never* mix the two together), wipe down the walls and surfaces of all the furniture. Have the carpets and upholstery cleaned. The same measures must be taken in the family car as well.

Don't buy an air filter with the idea it is going to make your cigarettes smokeless. *Don't replace carpeting with hardwood floors* with the idea that one expensive effort compensates for your expensive and unhealthy habit. *Don't move to Arizona* or change doctors if you are not willing to make some changes in your own life.

No, I don't have "No Smoking" tattooed on my forehead, and I've never spoken out on smoking before writing this book. I have been mildly victimized by it in the past, but I am a big girl and I can walk away from those whose smoke irritates me. My daughter cannot. If we are sitting in a restaurant or seated on a plane and someone lights a cigarette, the same amount of smoke that irritates my nose irritates my daughter's. With her allergies and sinus problems, the lining of her nose becomes irritated. Her sinus drain ports swell and become a cesspool of infection. The infection in turn feeds the asthma and guess who suffers? An innocent victim and her family.

There is no controversy surrounding this subject. You have the most to gain by making a commitment to cleaning up the air that your child breathes.

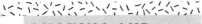

SMOKING AND ASTHMA

There have been a number of studies on the effect of parental smoking on the respiratory health of their children. Most studies demonstrate increased respiratory illness in the children of smokers, especially during the first two years of life. Tracheitis (inflammation of the trachea) and bronchitis occur significantly more frequently in infants exposed to cigarette smoke in the home.

A study by Doctors F. A. Pedreira, V. L. Guandolo, E. J. Feroli, et al. reported in *Pediatrics* 1985; 75:594 showed that a smoking mother imposes greater risks on the infant than a smoking father. For children beyond the age of infancy, when the mother smoked the children suffered 20 to 35 percent more respiratory problems such as wheezing, coughing and bronchitis compared with children living in homes without smokers. Illness and symptom frequencies were directly related to the number of cigarettes smoked by the child's mother.

Smokers contaminate their

WOOD AND COAL STOVES

If your home is designed to rely on an alternative heat source such as wood or coal, purchase only *airtight* wood and coal stoves. Airtight coal stoves are not as dirty as those used in the old days and are very efficient producers of heat. Kerosene heaters are not recommended.

Well-insulated homes almost always increase the potency of all indoor pollutants, including smoke. To minimize indoor pollution, install a catalytic converter (a device which burns the smoke given off by the logs). Ask your stove dealer about this. Wood should never be stored in the house. Clean up any dirt or debris that falls off the wood when you load it into the stove.

Other tips:

• Don't burn the wood or

clothes, their cars, their hair, etc., with very powerful irritants, which may cause problems for the person with asthma even if he is not exposed to the smoke itself.—Debbie Scherrer

coal with the stove door open.

• Enclose the fireplace with airtight doors, which are kept closed while the fire is burning.

• Once you get the fire burning, feed it with large chunks of hardwood. Avoid soft pines or poplars, twigs or green (unseasoned) wood.

• You can order a device called the Quantum Eye, which measures the amount of carbon monoxide released by your stove into the air of your home, for about $10. The address is in the Resources section of this book.

• Use a humidifier or keep a kettle of water on the stove to replenish some of the moisture in the air. Coal- and wood-burning stoves dry the air, which is not good for asthmatics.

PETS

We recently said tearful goodbyes to a dear member of our family, Tasha. Had Tasha lived, she would have been fifteen years old in two more months, pretty old for a German Shepherd mix.

I'd only known her for the last eleven years. Dale rescued her from the pound in his college years. When Dale and I met, he was a bachelor living with a dog in a condo and I was a widow living in a house with two small children. When we married, Tasha was part of the vows and as I look back over the years, I can't say I ever regretted it.

However, there was a time a few years ago when I feared we faced a decision between Tasha and Brooke. It should seem like such a simple choice. A child is worth far more than a hound. In the process of trying to rid our home of any possible allergens that might be affecting Brooke, we found a new home on a farm for Tasha where we were *sure* she'd be happy. After three months, her new owner called us to say Tasha was dying of a broken heart. She had refused to eat and would not get up even to walk around. The new owner said Tasha was so weak she did not expect the dog to live.

Dale and I hopped in the car and drove out to see her. As soon as Tasha saw us, she leaped to her feet and ran over, jumping up and licking our faces. With very mixed feelings we took her home, where she regained her weight and coat luster quickly.

After weighing the options, we knew that to send Tasha away would be to send her to a premature death. To do this without really knowing if Brooke's asthma and allergies would improve was more than we could justify. It was a problem with no clear solution we could live with so we found a compromise. Tasha was not to sleep in Brooke's room (though Brooke secretly encouraged it on more than one occasion), and Tasha was to be bathed frequently and kept outside as much as possible.

We never did have any conclusive evidence that Brooke was allergic to dogs. We *knew* how she reacted around cats, birds and horses. It was quite obvious she was allergic to these animals. But to dogs, we saw no decrease in peak flow readings or outward sign of allergy or asthma, even if she put her face on the animal. Her asthma and allergies had not changed for the better while Tasha was gone, even though we had cleaned our home thoroughly.

Had we known conclusively that Brooke was allergic to Tasha, as painful as it would have been we could not have brought Tasha back home. We had two birds, finches, when Brooke was born. We had them for almost two years before we realized her facial rash was an allergic response to them. As soon as we knew it, we found the birds a new home.

A cat tried to adopt us once but as soon as Brooke broke out in hives and started wheezing, we abandoned that idea and took the stray to the shelter.

Pets! They do manage to work their way into our lives. Unfortunately, pets often create problems with no easy answers when they concern the allergic child.

Here are a few ground rules concerning pets and allergic or asthmatic family members:

- If you don't have a pet and can live without one, try to do it.

- If you cannot live without a pet, try something like tropical fish or goldfish, lizards or even snakes. I am not wild about the last two, but with three boys in the house, we've had our share of the critters.

- Cats or dogs with short hair are just as much of a problem for allergic people as breeds with long hair. There is no such thing as a nonallergic breed of dog.

- Animal fur is not the problem. Dander and outdoor allergens such as pollens and molds that cling to the fur are the real culprits. Another problem is the animal proteins found in saliva and urine.

• If your child has an asthma attack or breaks out in hives or a rash every time he is near or touches a particular animal, that is positive proof of an allergy either to the animal itself or to the pollen or mold spores that cling to the fur. Avoidance of the allergen is the best solution even if it means finding a new home for the pet.

• If you already own a pet and you suspect an allergy, ask your doctor to test your child for allergy to your pet. If the skin test is positive, find a temporary home for your pet, vacuum and clean the house and see if the asthma improves. Give the trial period at least eight to twelve weeks because for many children, asthma and allergies tend to run in cycles. (The child is sick for two weeks, then well for four weeks, and so on.)

• If you are faced with a situation that has no clear solution, such as ours, make sure you keep the pet out of the house or apartment as much as possible and absolutely, positively, keep the pet out of the child's room. Also, expect to take some heat from people who think that all people who have real allergies can't have pets. Believe me, I've had my share of explaining to do.

• The majority of people who test negative to a specific animal are not allergic to it. However, a small percentage of people who test negative to cat or dog are in fact very allergic! The proof is in the pudding, so they say. If you test negative to cat or dog but have asthma or allergy symptoms upon exposure, you are allergic.

• If you must find a new home for a pet, do not explain the ordeal to the children as "getting rid of" something like old tennis shoes. Equally important is to avoid making one child the reason that the family must give up the pet.

There is no best way to explain this unpleasant prospect because each family has its own special circumstances. Even if Mom or Dad has to be the bad guy, it is better than inflicting that role on a child who is no more able to change the facts of his allergy than change the weather.

• If you have a pet and it makes your child wheeze, sneeze or otherwise uncomfortable, the rights of the child to breathe must come first! Don't complain about how life is so terrible with asthma if you are unwilling to assess realistically the value of the lives of those you've been entrusted to raise. I know many people who brag that they are allergic to their pet. Don't fall into the trap of believing that a house is not a home unless there's a dog or some other furry animal to come home to at the end of the day.

• Some doctors recommend that if you presently do not have a dog or cat that it would be wise not to get one, even if the child tests negative for animals. This is because allergies have a tendency to develop with exposure over a period of time, and it is quite possible that while your family's love and attachment to the animal grow, an allergic reaction may be developing. It is easy to say, "We'll try it, and we'll just get rid of the pet if it starts to cause a problem," but the reality is that by the time the allergy is manifested, the animal will have become a member of the family and the separation will be painful. Thus, it may be wise to avoid this potential problem.

• A furry animal can cause problems for a pollen-sensitive child even if the child is not allergic to the animal itself. When a dog or cat goes outside, its fur can collect large amounts of pollens, which are then brought into the house when the animal comes in.

There is hope that new medications will become available that will enable allergy sufferers to have pets. One new drug, CI-949, is being tested for its ability to reduce delayed symptoms of asthma caused by cat protein. Dr. Richard Rosenthal, Chief of the Allergy Section at Fairfax Hospital, Fairfax, VA, assistant professor at Johns Hopkins School of Medicine, Baltimore, MD., and one of the investigators of the drug, states that cat dander is the most allergenic of all animal danders and affects millions of Americans. Cat allergy symptoms range from itchy, watery eyes to sneezing, shortness of breath and hives. Some people, particularly those who have asthma, will experience delayed respiratory symptoms up to twelve hours later. The medication is targeted 'at this reaction. Also, immunotherapy does calm allergic reactions to some pets, the greatest success being with dogs.

We will miss Tasha and the joy she brought to our home. There is no easy way to deal with the loss of a pet whether it has been taken from your home by its death or your child's allergy. The day we said goodbye to Tasha, we each took turns hugging her. Brooke flung her arms around our dying Tasha's neck and nuzzled her face against the dog's. Brooke lingered, muffling her sobs deep in Tasha's fur. I cringed, thinking if she didn't have an asthma attack after this, we could be certain that she had never been allergic to Tasha in the first place. As I leaned forward to comfort Brooke, I noticed that Tasha had tears in her eyes too.

Brooke continued to cry into the evening but no asthma or indication of allergies or wheezing followed. With time, I know that my family will want another dog. We have agreed to wait one year to see if Brooke's allergies improve as the result of no pets in the family. Brooke understands the agreement but will not shoulder the blame if we don't get another dog. I will gladly carry that burden for her.

FOOD ALLERGIES

If your current methods of asthma management don't deliver the expected results and you have never considered food allergies, it may be time to investigate the foods your child eats.

Some doctors don't test for food allergies simply because they don't feel the tests are reliable. False diagnosis of food allergies often results from such tests as radionics, radiesthesia, radionic ecology, radionic hair testing, pulse testing, leucocyte cytotoxicity and hair trace metal analysis.

While no testing method is completely accurate, there are skin tests that can provide a basis from which to develop a diet for the child suspected of having food allergies. The tests' results, when combined with parental observation, can provide valuable information which can substantially reduce the incidence of asthma.

Food allergies can be revealed in more ways than just asthma. Skin conditions such as hives, eczema and atopic dermatitis (inflammation of the skin) are frequently symptoms of food allergies. Some of the common offenders are eggs, milk, peanuts, fish, shellfish and strawberries. Less frequent offenders are yeast, food additives, azo dyes and benzoate preservatives. Allergy to cow's milk, eggs, soy, gluten, brown rice, chicken and fish can produce symptoms of stomach and bowel disorders. Even migraine headaches have on occasion been connected to a particular food.

Children with food allergies often require a special menu that can differ drastically from the traditional American menu. For example, tuna salad sandwiches just aren't tuna salad sandwiches if you take the mayo out. The celery, pickles and tuna simply don't hold together without a little glue! Bottled salad dressing would be a good substitute but most are made with ingredients to which Brooke is allergic, so we opt for tuna salad on the plate with bread on the side. Otherwise, when she bites into the sandwich, it would be anybody's guess whether she'd get any tuna before it tumbled out the other end.

I will never forget when the allergist told us how severe her reactions to the tests were. Then he told us what she *could* eat because that was easier than telling us what she *couldn't* eat. In Brooke's case, the skin testing was pretty accurate.

At first I had to fight the urge to feel sorry for Brooke. But when I realized that even with her limited diet, she could still eat a more healthful variety of food than many children in the world, I had to be thankful for the foods she could eat.

I wish I could say that ridding her diet of offending foods also rid her of asthma. It did help noticeably and did clear her skin and reduced the incidence of hives but she still had asthma. Some children respond so well to special diets that they rarely require medication for asthma.

Brooke has never really objected to her special diet. She has grown up on it and really doesn't know any different. But there have been times when we sat down to the table to thank the Lord for our food when the "amen" was followed by, "Brooke, I am so sorry! I forgot your dinner! I'll get it." She smiles, forgives me and supplies dinner conversation over her empty plate while I pop her meal into the microwave!

HERE ARE SOME TIPS FOR PARENTS WITH KIDS ON A DIFFERENT DIET FROM THE REST OF THE FAMILY:

- Buy individual serving sizes of canned foods and keep them on the pantry shelf.

- Allow your child to make menu choices. "Would you like lamb burgers or turkey cutlets tonight?" "Neither" is not an acceptable answer.

- Try to incorporate "look-alike" foods in your child's diet. If the family is having hamburgers and your child is allergic to beef, grill a lamb burger instead. When eating spaghetti, serve it without meat to a child who cannot tolerate meat.

- Do not preface serving a special meal with negative comments like, "I am sorry you have to eat this" or "I wish you could eat what we have." And don't let siblings act the way siblings often do by casting a contorted glance at the special meal and making comments like, "Ooh, gross—apple juice on Cheerios!"

- Multivitamin supplements and additional calcium (especially if the child is allergic to milk) can be helpful if your child's diet is unbalanced. However, read the labels as some vitamins contain dyes, binders and flavorings to which your child may be sensitive.

- If you have a food-allergic child, identify "safe" foods in your freezer or pantry with a blue dot label or some other kind of sticker. This way, baby-sitters won't make the mistake of giving your child a forbidden food.

Special diets do require a little extra work but don't undo the good of the diet by making the child feel guilty for causing you the inconvenience. By having a proper attitude, you teach your child by example to give of him or herself unselfishly. After all, your child would do the same for you if called upon. Who knows, someday, they may be.

MILK

Milk has been identified as a potential trigger of asthma and/or allergy symptoms, although the actual physiology of the reaction is not completely understood. All we as parents know is that some of us observe reportable symptoms that can be relieved when the milk (or other offending food) is removed from the diet.

Some Hidden Sources of Milk

Au gratin foods
Baked goods
Butter
Candy
Casein, caseinate or sodium caseinate (listed on labels)
Cheese
Chocolate
Cold cuts
Creamed or scalloped vegetables or other foods

Creamed soups
Curds
Frankfurters and bologna
Gravy
Ice cream
Malted milk
Margarine
Milk Sherbet
Pudding
Salad dressings
Waffle, pancake and biscuit mixes
Whey
White sauces

—From the *Isomil Cookbook* by Ross Laboratories, Columbus, Ohio.

Some children who are milk-sensitive or allergic can use nondairy products, but even these products can cause severe problems for some children if they contain even one milk product or protein. Read labels, check the ingredients!

I recently learned through a letter from Stanislaus Ting, M.D., an allergist in Las Cruces, New Mexico, of a product which gives the impression that it is especially made for people with milk allergy or milk intolerance, when in truth it can actually cause a life-threatening reaction in a small percentage of unsuspecting milk-allergic individuals.

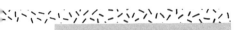

LOVING RECIPES

My three-year-old son has asthma and multiple food allergies. For his first birthday I built a graham cracker cake using graham crackers and apple butter. He loved it—as did his friends. —Mother in Fairfax, Virginia

I received a quick muffin or bread recipe from the Canadian

The product is advertised as a replacement for milk in the diet and is being marketed directly to doctors for their patients. Although the product does contain milk protein, this company calls its product "Vitamite Lactose Free Non-Dairy Beverage." Dr. Ting reported to the makers of Vitamite an incident that involved an eight-month-old boy with known milk allergy who sustained a life-threatening reaction to their product. The company, Diehl Specialties International, has agreed to put a warning label on each container which reads, "Contains milk protein. Not recommended for people with milk allergy. Consult your physician."

Allergy Society for those with allergies to milk and eggs. Use Duncan Hines banana bread mix. Instead of the egg, add 40 ml (a scant 3 tablespoons) of safflower oil. I always add an extra banana for thickening but the original recipe did not call for it.—Mother in Woodbridge, Virginia

There are other "nondairy" products which include milk protein, although these do not advertise that they can be used safely by milk-sensitive people. So read labels!

SULFITES

Sulfite-sensitive people can use a product called Sulfitest made by Center Laboratories to home-test food products for sulfites. The FDA estimates that the preservative is contained in 1,100 marketed drugs, all of which are now required to carry a warning.

SOY

Most of today's processed foods contain soy because it is an inexpensive source of protein. Sometimes I wonder if the increase in food allergies isn't due to the fact that our food products have so many added things in them. Years ago you didn't need to worry that salad dressings or cookies would have soy in them. If soy is a problem for your child, watch labeling carefully. Some labels state: "This product may contain one or more of the following oils: soy, cottonseed, palm kernel . . ." If your child is particularly sensitive to soy, you may have to begin baking your own cookies to avoid it.

BIRTHDAY PARTIES UNLIMITED

A birthday isn't a birthday without a party. But planning festivities for a child with food allergies and his friends can be quite a challenge.

My knowledge of how to do it has been acquired through trial and error—with lots of error! There was the memorable year we tried a new chocolate cake recipe. It was egg-less, wheatless and eat-less. It flowed out of the cake pan and ignited as it cascaded to

LIVING WITH THE FOOD-ALLERGIC CHILD

Food allergies can be a mild nuisance or severe and life-threatening. One mother wrote that if she was given the opportunity to rid her child of asthma or food allergies, she wouldn't know which one to choose. Another mother, a teacher, called me to say that her child is so allergic to certain food products that making meals without accidentally contaminating her child's food is very stressful (not to mention all the extra cooking and serving utensils she must use).

Sometimes allergic reactions to foods are so bizarre that other people find it hard to believe that the parent is not simply fabricating a story. For example, Brooke wanted to taste a piece of shrimp one time so I gave her a piece no larger than a baby pea. Within minutes she broke out in hives and started wheezing. Most of her food allergies are easy to control or adapt to even though there are very few foods she can eat. However, there are children who have similar, if not even more severe, reactions to foods than Brooke did with the shrimp.

Jelly can be easily contaminated with peanut butter or milk proteins (from butter) and cause problems for a child who is allergic to either of these products. I know mothers who purchase special bread, bagels, butcher cuts of meat and lunch meats from a

the oven floor. It looked like one of those snakes the kids buy for the Fourth of July. We were in a pinch to take the cake to a party so we drilled a hole in what was left of it with a shish-kebab skewer, threw in a candle and vowed to laugh about it . . . the next day!

Then there was the fall I made a popcorn and gumdrop cake. Shane, my allergic son, was three and I can still remember all those darling munchkins drooling as they tried to eat the cake that was truly a tooth fairy's dream.

Well, the joke cakes are over (let's hope), and we discovered 101 ways to make Rice Krispies bars into birthday treats. We have colored them in several shades and layered them, rolled them out and cut them with metal cookie cutters and even molded them onto popsicle sticks. We've also added chocolate chips, raisins, sunflower nuts and M&M's—always to the kids' delight.

Now Shane can have ice cream, but in our no-milk diet days he would have Baskin-Robbins ice (sherbet has milk). Our biggest success was to cover the bottom of a springform pan with a doily, attach the rim and then layer different flavors of softened Baskin-Rob-

bins ice with chocolate sauce, butterscotch or marshmallow cream. The springform pan makes molding foolproof and the finished product looks like a real cake.—Nancy Carol Sanker, President of Asthmatic/Allergic Children in Fort Collins, Colorado

local bakery or butcher shop because they know that the owner will wash his equipment before slicing their purchase. This way, he avoids contaminating their food with foods recently cut on the machine. Though making an extra stop at the deli or the butcher shop may seem a little extreme, some children's lives depend on it.

Check the Resources section of this book for more information on food allergies and where to find help.

GROWING UP WITH ASTHMA

Parents make many adjustments during the period between diagnosis and control, and these changes can affect every aspect of parenting. From diapers to dating, at school and at play, asthma travels with our children. And asthma is a family affair.

Part II will focus on the practical side of parenting our special children as they grow up with asthma. Don't count on your child "growing out of asthma." Be prepared, accept the challenge before you *and* your child and then be thankful for the respite if it comes.

P A R T

II

CHAPTER 8

FROM
DIAPERS TO
DATING

ASTHMA AFFECTS EACH STAGE OF CHILDHOOD
differently. In this chapter, you'll learn about managing
asthma at each age—including special tools of the trade, triggers and early warning signals, medications, self-management skills and other tips.

BIRTH TO AGE TWO

Many children with asthma seem almost to have been born wheezing. After assembling all the data, initiating therapies and ruling out possible causes for the breathing difficulties, the doctors were left with the diagnosis of asthma. This diagnosis often marks the beginning of what many parents describe as the most frustrating period in asthma management.

Although we love our babies, we are many times unprepared for the exhausting responsibility of caring for them, especially when they have a chronic illness such as asthma. We expect caring for a newborn to revolve around interpreting cries, frequent feedings and changing diapers. We do not expect to watch our babies struggle to breathe, to spend days and nights in the hospital or take what may appear to be large amounts of medicine.

An asthma baby's list of firsts (first smile, first step, first tooth) often includes such items as: first breathing treatment, first hospitalization, first ride in the ambulance. The nursery becomes an infirmary of vaporizers, medicines and creams. To complicate things further, babies with asthma frequently have eczema or skin rashes that make them less than picture-perfect.

Family and friends often do not know how to respond. They offer advice, some good, but much unintentionally hurtful. Suddenly, you may be scolded for spoiling your baby, holding him too much or nursing instead of bottle-feeding (or vice versa).

One mother wrote that she was tired of people dissecting her marriage to find out why her infant son had asthma. Some of your family members or friends may shrug off the severity of the disease by saying things like, "No one ever dies from asthma anymore" or "Don't worry, she'll probably outgrow it." Others think there's a psychological stigma associated with the disease so they deny asthma's existence by calling it something else. Some adult asthmatics even go so far as to advise, "Just leave him alone and he'll do fine. I survived, didn't I?"

Asthma in infants can be more frightening than in older children because often we don't know they are having trouble until the attack has advanced. Their lungs are so tiny that it doesn't take much to obstruct them dangerously. As the child grows older and is able to communicate, and as you become more familiar with the early warning signals and triggers, the frequency and severity of the asthma should improve.

Do not confuse controlling asthma with "growing out of asthma." With controlled asthma, the disease is still present but well managed. Infants and toddlers with asthma triggered by only viral infections are the best candidates for remission of symptoms. As the child's immune system matures and the size of the airways increases, the frequency and severity of asthma improves as well. Be aware, however, that some of these babies will develop allergen-triggered asthma as they grow older.

Even though your baby is young, your doctor should prepare you to handle each stage of your child's asthma. You should have a treatment plan for early intervention

OVERPROTECTIVE?

I have a nineteen-month-old son who has had asthma since he was about nine months old.

He has been in the hospital several times and has had pneumonia and other serious viral infections. His immune system is weak and he catches colds and flu everytime he turns around. Of course, this sends him into bronchial spasm, which requires at least two doctor's visits, at least two weeks of theophylline, maybe a few days of steroids and several injections of adrenalin. He also has his nebulizer treatments three times a day. And let's not forget the plain misery of all this for him!

So as a result, I have to be very careful who my son plays with or is exposed to. I had to stop bringing him to the nursery on Sunday at church, (thank God I am home with him during the week) and I have to be careful that his friends or cousins aren't sick before he can see them.

My problem is that some people understand and some people don't. I have to stress to my friends that I don't consider my son better or too good to play with their children but the facts are that he gets sick very easily. One child's sniffle is my child's asthma!

I have been round and round with my mother-in-law, who

when an attack is approaching. You should know what to do in case the first medications given do not bring about the desired results. You should know when to take your baby to the doctor or emergency room.

Though this time of your life may seem very stressful, use it as an opportunity to grow closer to those around you. Rally the support of other family members, especially other siblings. Don't let it destroy you.

One mom wrote:

I have a sixteen-month-old who has been hospitalized twice for asthma and, of course, there have been additional trips to the emergency room and the doctor's office. When he is well, it is like heaven. He is so happy, active and alert. But when he is sick, our whole world is turned upside down. My husband and I are still trying to cope with the stresses of living with an asthmatic and the fears of the next attack. *We want to be "good" asthma parents and hope that we can learn to control it without those scary trips to the hospital. We have a wonderful son and know that someday asthma will be something we will be able to deal with.*

This mother's sentiments are echoed almost every day. Though you may many times feel isolated and lonely, you are *not* alone. And in time, you will be coping far better than you ever expected.

Tools of the Trade

Some infants benefit from the use of a home nebulizer. Your doctor is the best judge of your child's need for a nebulizer and will show you how to use one.

thinks I am totally wrong for keeping Ashton away from other children. We have actually had arguments about this. More than once!

I have done a lot of research, and I question my excellent pediatrician endlessly about all of this. I feel that I am well informed and know what is best for my child. Other people see me as overprotective and finicky even after I explain things to them. This is the most frustrating thing for me.

Just recently, cold and flu season having passed, I have let my son play with other children and we will take swim classes soon. I realize that it would be cruel to isolate him completely from other kids. Right now I'm holding my breath (no pun intended) and praying that he won't catch another virus.—Mother in Cape Coral, Florida

One of the most useful tools for most parents of infants who have asthma is a stethoscope. Ask your doctor to teach you how to use a stethoscope.

· · ·

Early Warning Signals

Early warning signals are clues that alert you to an impending attack. It may be difficult to determine your baby's specific signals until she has had several attacks. It is not always easy to tell what differentiates "normal" crabby behavior due to teething, "terrible twos" and a host of other causes from behavior caused by the child's not feeling well, medication side effects, etc. *Write things down.* Keep a daily diary of symptoms, suspected early warning signals (no matter how obscure), suspected triggers and medications given and their results. Over time you will begin to see a pattern.

Some *early warning signals* you may notice are:

- A sudden change in sleeping habits
- A runny yellowish or green mucus from the nose
- Bluish or light purple rings under the child's eyes
- Swollen face
- Slight cough
- A sudden change in behavior, i.e., less active, short spurts of energy, irritability
- Pale complexion
- Restless, fitful sleep
- Excessive drooling

Signs of an Attack

Signals that accompany an *attack already in progress* and require immediate medical treatment are:

- The baby is wheezing audibly (high-pitched sounds).
- The skin pulls in around the ribs and at the dip in the collarbone with each breath (called chest retraction).
- The baby's stomach heaves with each breath in an effort to force air out of the lungs.
- The baby's fingernails or lips have lost their pink color and are now purplish or blue.
- The baby's skin color is dusky (gray if child is Caucasian, a blanched version of the child's normal skin color if child is black or Oriental).
- The baby cannot stop coughing and his eyes appear to bug out of their sockets with each cough.
- The baby is exhausted.
- The baby is not voiding normally.
- The baby is resisting nourishment.
- The baby's breaths are rapid and shallow. The number of breaths or respirations per minute should be 20 to 30 in infants and 15 to 25 in toddlers during sleep. Respirations per minute are more rapid when awake, averaging 60 in infants and 35 in toddlers.

If you see any of the above signals, get immediate medical attention for your baby!

Triggers

Some allergic triggers to consider are:

- Pets, especially indoor pets such as dogs, cats and birds
- House dust and dust mites (stuffed animals included)

- Molds and fungi (in air vents, on walls, in window frames, rotting leaves, humidifiers, diaper pails)
- Airborne pollens (those plants and trees that are wind pollinated)
- Foods

Some nonallergic triggers to consider:

- Temperature and barometric pressure changes—even when your child stays inside the house
- Smoke, including all tobacco smoke
- Odors, perfumes, cleaning chemicals, deodorants, hair spray, paint
- Humidity levels
- Laundry detergents and drier "softener sheets"
- Exercise
- Colds, viruses, bacteria
- Laughing and/or crying
- Gastroesophageal reflux (stomach acids seep back up into and irritate the esophagus and/or are inhaled into the lungs)
- Teething

Medications

Some of the medicines your baby must take relax the twitchy bronchial muscles that are wrapped around his airways. These medicines may include bronchodilators. Another medication which your baby may need is a steroid, an anti-inflammatory drug. Sometimes other medications such as decongestants and antihistamines are added.

Frequently, parents are alarmed at their baby's behavior after taking medications. Sometimes babies become more lively and active. Other babies cry more frequently, are more sensitive to noise or cannot sleep. These changes in behavior can many times be traced to the side effects of one or more of the medications.

As babies grow into the toddler stage, your efforts to keep your chemically stimulated child from "bouncing off the walls" may literally wear you out. Many parents have noted that their wee ones keep moving until they are drained of energy and then they crash.

Report any excessive crying, stomach cramps, excessive jitteriness, vomiting or difficulty in waking your child. Obviously, some of these symptoms could be related to a medical problem other than medication, but they should be reported to your doctor in case a change of instruction would help. If you are still concerned about the medications your baby must take or the therapy your doctor has prescribed, get a second opinion from another good doctor. Side effects are not the only alternatives we have to coughing and wheezing children anymore.

Child Care

Day care centers, play groups, church nurseries and mother's day out programs can expose your child to a lot of germs. The greater the number of children, the greater number of germs the child is likely to pick up. Don't forget that babies are famous for teething on whatever is handy. Teething items are often inadvertently shared, so the germs are too. Finding an individual baby-sitter with no other children *may* reduce the incidence of germ sharing.

Church nurseries can fuel the colds that flare on Tuesday, Wednesday and Thursday, start to get better on Friday and clear up enough by Sunday that the baby looks healthy enough to take to church again. Many church nurseries have strict rules about toys, strollers, walkers and cribs. Our nursery provides clean bedding each time an infant is put into a crib. The automatic swings are kept clean and all toys and bedding are washed by a volunteer each week. Some parents have been known to provide their own walker and stroller and request that nursery volunteers do not place other children in their equipment because they are trying to reduce exposure to germs.

I could not put Brooke into a play school setting until she was about three years old because she was so susceptible to colds. Fortunately, I found another mother who would trade days of the week with me, and we would swap taking care of each other's kids. She understood the "germ situation" and did not take offense. Fortunately, as babies get older their tolerance for colds and viruses usually improves.

Be forewarned that others may view you as overprotective and maybe even a little wacky. The less you say about the problem, the less likely they are to notice. If a confrontation is unavoidable, state the facts and ask for their compassion and understanding.

In interviewing potential baby-sitters, you are looking for a nonsmoking person who preferably will come into your home. If that is not possible, her home should be clean and have no smokers; it should also be free of pets known or suspected to cause allergies. There is no need to offend prospective baby-sitters by insisting they change their living habits. Simply weave questions concerning the health needs of your child into the interview and if they are not answered adequately, you need to interview someone else.

Ideally, all sitters should be as attentive as Mickey McCarthy, who wrote the following article for *MA Report:*

I have recently had the opportunity to care for several children with asthma and severe allergies. Keeping children overnight is always a big responsibility but these children take a little extra care. Here are some of the things I have found important to take care of ahead of time.

Make sure you understand the child's health problem. It is so important to know what to look for and how to handle calmly any problem that may arise.

Explain the health condition of the baby to all family members. We had one baby who could not eat any "regular" food, so I had to make sure my girls did not "share" their goodies. (Often little ones cannot remember which things they are allergic to so it is best if everyone understands all food must be okayed first.) If you explain asthma to your family they will alert you to any unusual breathing or behavior. It is good to explain that the child may take lots of medicine and/or breathing treatments.

Get written permission to seek and sign for medical help in case of an emergency. Find out what your local area requires to make it legally binding (such as witnesses or notarized), then have the child's parents sign the paper as well as yourself. You should both have copies.

Have a list containing the name, address and phone number of the child's doctor. If the child is on immunotherapy (shots), know when the last one was given. If the child is on medication, I have found it helpful to set the alarm. Mom remembers as it is her daily routine but it is not mine and I would feel awful if the child had even a mild attack simply because I forgot to give the

*medication on time. I always like to have written in-
structions for medication and diet to refer to as needed.*

*I cleaned the curtains, dusted and vacuumed the
sleeping area thoroughly the night before the child arrived. Be sure to remove plants (if necessary) a few days
ahead.*

*Check and see if the child needs special soaps for
bathing or for laundry. We also washed the dog; however she is outside mostly.*

*I have three daughters and they often get quite excited
when we have visitors overnight. Even so, it is important for the child with asthma to stay on his or her
normal routine, or at least get enough sleep.*

*Ask any and all questions you have of the parents
even if you feel they are silly. The more you understand
the better prepared you will be and the more confident
the parents will be to leave their little one.*

*I have enjoyed having these little visitors in my home.
It is a little extra work and care but it isn't hard and
certainly worth the effort.—Mickey McCarthy, Manas-
sas, Virginia*

You should be warned that many child care givers do not
want to take responsibility for a baby with health problems.
If your initial interview reveals someone who meets your
standards, you must tell her about your baby's health care
requirements. If she seems frightened or unwilling to become part of your baby's health care team, you need to continue your search.

Sometimes grandparents become involved in the care of a
baby so that both parents can work. It is certainly a relief for
parents when they have someone who has a true interest in
the needs of the baby.

Whoever takes care of your child should be willing to medicate, take the child to the doctor in case of emergency, report suspected medication side effects, be able to determine if medication is not acting as expected, avoid triggers and be aware of early warning signals. You should not expect the baby-sitter to take your baby for well visits or allergy shots unless you have discussed this specifically ahead of time.

Remember, the responsibility for learning appropriate asthma management techniques and teaching them to others is *yours.* Whether your child care needs are filled by a day care center or a professional nanny, you must enable the person responsible to respond appropriately to even the worst scenarios or the consequences could be severe.

Timely Tips

• If your doctor recommends using a humidifier in the baby's room during the dry, winter months, don't shut the door completely as too much humidity can build up and the baby can become chilled when brought to another room. You should not see or feel condensation on the crib or walls but you may see some on the windows. Follow the instructions that came with the humidifier to control the amount of humidity produced.

   Many people prefer cool-mist humidifiers to the steam vaporizers or vice versa. If your doctor recommends one, ask which one he or she uses or believes is best. Humidifiers go on sale late winter to early spring. Watch for store sales.

   Humidifiers and vaporizers are excellent breeders of molds and bacteria. Follow the instructions for cleaning that came with the unit. When in continuous use, vaporizers should be cleaned daily.

- When packing the diaper bag, besides the usual stash of diapers and clothes, include any scheduled medications, your stethoscope and emergency care information. Pack your diaper bag carefully each time you leave the house. If other siblings prone to exploration are around, keep the bag out of reach. One mom laminated an emergency care card to the back of her child's car seat just in case she was involved in an automobile wreck and was not able to give appropriate medical information at the scene. Though this may seem extreme to some people, you will know if your child's case warrants this kind of action.

- Environmental controls may have been prescribed by your doctor. The most important ones involve the removal of stuffed animals and toys and unnecessary room clutter. Though the measures seem harsh at first, take the precautions and see if there is an improvement. Replace regular stuffed animals with those made specifically for allergy patients (see Resources section) or those that can be machine washed easily. (Avoid washing too many stuffed animals at once. It cost us a new pump on our washing machine to learn this one the hard way.) Cotton curtains for the baby's room are okay if you will remember to wash them frequently. Otherwise, bright roll-up shades make a healthy alternative.

- Avoid using baby powder unless absolutely necessary as the fine particles of dust are breathed into baby's lungs. (This is true for nonallergic babies, too.)

- Asthma in infants is characterized by rapid, shallow breathing. This increases your baby's need for fluids. During episodes of wheezing, provide extra clear fluids (such as flat 7UP or caffeine-free cola, Jell-O water, apple juice or water). Be careful about too much apple juice or the baby may get loose stools. Avoid caffeine. At this point, unless sugar is a problem for your baby, don't feel guilty about giving your baby the soda. Because your baby is not feeling well, she probably is not eating properly and will need the extra calories. The important thing is to get lots of liquids into your baby.

- Breast milk is the best nourishment for most infants with a family history of asthma and allergies. Several studies have shown that breast feeding may actually reduce the liklihood of allergies developing. It is also suggested that nursing mothers avoid foods commonly associated with allergies. Do not be in too big a hurry to begin starting foods. Follow your doctor's instructions and when you do start, do it slowly, adding only one new food per week and watching carefully for a reaction.

- Adults love to give little ones finger foods. This is particularly true at adult parties and family gatherings. If your baby is food allergic, avoid taking him to such parties or make sure you keep your eyes open. Do not allow people to grab your baby out of your arms unless you are smiling when you say, "Michael is yours for the moment but only if you don't let him eat anything you don't clear with me first." It may help if you provide your own finger foods for your baby. Even so, make it clear that under no circumstances should the baby be allowed to eat anything unless it has been cleared first with you. If people need an explanation, make it simple and direct and say it with a sincere though serious smile (another neat trick!): "Michael has severe food allergies which are potentially life-threatening." They may decide to hand your baby back, but so what.

- When introducing medical ideas to a toddler, it sometimes helps if a favorite baby doll gets a "breathing treatment" or an allergy shot first. Boys are just as accepting of this idea as girls at this age.

- Keep a *written* list of known or suspected early warning signals and food and environmental triggers in a convenient place for easy referral.

- If one of your children has allergies, there is a chance that your other babies may, also. Take extra precautions right from the start, making the new baby's room as allergen-free as that of your allergic child.

AGES THREE TO SIX

Despite our concerns over their coughs, colds and wheezing, our wee ones are growing up. They like nursery rhymes, fairy tales, building blocks and pretending. They are just like every other child their age except interwoven into their lives are breathing treatments, medications, allergy-free treats and environmental controls.

Your child may be newly diagnosed with asthma or you may have gathered quite a library of information about the disease by this time. You understand asthma's potential to drive *you* crazy and that's why you are reading this book. You also want to know how to reduce asthma's impact on the physical and social development of your child.

The diagnosis of chronic asthma, be it mild, moderate or severe, establishes the ground rules. "Okay, my child has asthma. Where do we go from here?" The same old rules ap-

ply. You lessen asthma's impact when you prevent and control its symptoms.

Your first goal is to get asthma under control and keep it there. Your second goal is to enable your child gradually to accept responsibility for managing the asthma.

We *can* teach our children, especially at this young age, to adapt and adjust, to grow and explore, to react appropriately to their illness and to work to control it. When we teach them while they are young, controlling asthma later in life is no big deal.

Sometimes it takes creative parenting to motivate strong-willed children to adapt their behaviors. One mom, Cindy, wrote of her five-year-old son, Jonathan's, problem with hysteria at allergy testing sessions and the success they experienced using a behavior modification technique she'd read about in *Redbook*.

Jonathan was particularly fond of Transformer toys at the peak of their popularity. So Cindy made a deal with him. He could earn the favored toy by demonstrating proper behavior at the doctor's office. He had to overcome his fear, walk from the waiting room to the examination room, and receive the shot without trying to run away or fight his mother.

Cindy purchased a small spiral-bound notebook and a packet of stickers for Jonathan. Each time Jonathan accepted the tests or shots without losing control, he earned a sticker. He was allowed to cry or even scream if he felt the need, but only when the needle was touching him and only if he did not move his arm. When the ten numbered pages in the sticker book were filled, he would receive the Transformer. If he was unable to meet the criteria, he received credit on one of the bonus pages that did not count toward the agreement.

Though Jonathan did begin to lose control at the next appointment, Cindy and the nurse controlled him physically while calmly talking about the great Transformer he was trying to earn. This placated him and he received a sticker to put on the bonus page. The following weeks showed rapid improvement, and after a bit of scrambling to buy the ever popular Transformer, Cindy presented the toy to her very proud son after the tenth successful shot. The nurses and doctors praised him, and Jonathan felt good about himself.

Tools of the Trade

At age four, some children can start using *flow meters.* Children at this age are more likely to perform if the flow meter becomes part of a game.

Parents can make a game of blowing into a regular flow meter by placing colored dots along the meter's shaft. Try to encourage your child to make the meter arrow reach a certain color. You should always cheer for your child when he has blown into it correctly. As he gets older, the cheers will be replaced with praise like, "Good job, David! Let's write the numbers down on our chart!" When you go to visit the doctor next, let your child present his "flow meter record" to the doctor, who should in turn praise his effort as well as collect appropriate data. Use your flow meter to forecast episodes, monitor ongoing problems and determine if the child is capable of playing out of doors or participating in physical activities.

If your doctor has prescribed the use of an *inhaler,* follow her instructions for proper inhaling technique. Otherwise the medication is more likely to sit on the child's tongue or on the back of the throat. If you are unsure of your child's ability to use the inhaler effectively or you see no improvement after the inhaler is used, try a *spacer,* and help your child

inhale the medication over two or three inhalations as opposed to one sudden blast.

Nebulizer compressor treatments, administered at home according to doctor's instructions, have eliminated emergency
room visits for many children. According to studies and the
testimony of many parents, nebulizer treatments have also
reduced the number of unscheduled office visits and hospitalizations.

A *stethoscope* is still a must if asthma is a problem more
than twice a year. It is a minor expense well worth the effort.
As always, ask your doctor to show you how to use it.

Pillow and mattress encasings will be helpful if your child
is sensitive to dust mites.

Early Warning Signals and Triggers

Your child is now old enough to begin telling you when she
feels "tight." She is likely to describe the way she feels in
amusing, though strangely accurate ways. She may describe
feeling tight as feeling like someone wrapped rubber bands
around her chest or that a monster is squeezing her. Some
children have dreams that they are having an asthma attack
and when they wake up, they find that they are not dreaming
at all. Some children have nightmares, or begin scratching
their face or the underside of their chin before their attack.
Use the list in Chapter 2 and make a note of any early warning signals and triggers you have noticed.

Medications

Your child may now be old enough that your doctor may
recommend using nasal sprays (don't ever use any of them,
including over-the-counter medications, without your doc-

tor's specific instructions), inhalers, pills instead of liquids, and eye drops.

As always, keep all medications out of the reach of young children. Keep activated charcoal on hand for accidental theophylline overdose. Contact your physician or the Poison Control Center in your area for dosing instructions.

You may notice medication side effects such as sleepiness, hyperactivity, headaches, nausea, stomach cramping, nervousness, depression and altered behavior among others. If your child cannot tolerate a medication, another medication can often be substituted. A certain degree of jitteriness may be noted if your child is on numerous medications to halt an attack; however, contact your doctor if side effects persist or the asthma is not improving. Children on long-term preventive asthma medications should not be expected to live with long-term medication side effects. Such side effects are no longer a necessary evil for most asthmatics.

Self-Management Skills

Most three- and four-year-olds can be taught to:

- Swallow a pill
- Use a flow meter with help
- Use a spacer with help
- Use a nebulizer with help
- Use nasal sprays with help
- Describe how they feel
- Breathe slowly and deeply if having an attack
- Recognize a few triggers
- Recognize a few early warning signals
- Slowly sip water while concentrating on slower breathing

Five- and six-year-olds can add the following to the above list:

- Use an inhaler if prescribed by the doctor
- Help assemble nebulizer treatments
- Recognize the names of medicines
- Stay calm while having an attack but also seek help
- Recognize some food and environmental asthma triggers
- Use nasal sprays without help
- Participate in activities that build physical stamina

Timely Tips

- When your child has an asthma attack, remember to remain calm, quickly assess the severity of the attack, medicate according to a prearranged plan and call your child's doctor if you have any questions. Some asthma attacks are sudden and severe while others have a more subtle start (this can be demonstrated by the regular use of a peak flow meter).

- Our little ones can and should be taught to participate in family responsibilities even though they have asthma. Helping to clear the table, taking out the trash, folding towels and keeping their room clean can be part of their daily routine.

- When using steam vaporizers, medications, mercury glass thermometers, menthol rubs or creams, be certain to keep them out of reach of curious youngsters.

- Always secure your child in a car seat even and especially when in route to the doctor's office or hospital for emergency treatment. If you are afraid you won't make it to a hospital in time without using excessive speed, call a rescue squad.

- Children who have sudden life-threatening allergies and/or asthma are now old enough to wear MedAlert bracelets. Also, children who require daily *oral* corticosteroids (see Chapter 5) should have this information on a bracelet as well.

- Teach your child the names of her medications and why each is being given. Example: "Jennifer, this is your Proven-til syrup and it helps you to breathe more easily." Spice up your explanations with some creative expressions.

- This is a good age to incorporate children's books and workbooks on asthma into their lives. See Resources section for suggestions.

- Breathing exercises that teach your child how to slow breathing during an attack and to use that time to think about the next appropriate action are very worthwhile. However, breathing exercises should not be substituted for medications!

- Food allergies may be a trigger in your child's asthma. Skin testing for food allergies is not entirely accurate but it can supply valuable information to help develop a healthy diet for your child.

- Susan Carlson of Streamwood, Illinois, shares suggestions with *MA* readers from time to time and this is one of our favorites. When your child wants a food that contains an ingredient to which he's allergic, offer a choice of substitutes. "No, you can't have ice cream but you can have animal crackers, an apple or a popsicle." This way you can avoid making him feel cheated.

• This is the age of play groups and preschool, which can present their own set of problems. Most have daily snacks, birthday celebrations and other treats. If your child has food allergies, keep a supply of safe snacks at school so she will not be excluded from the fun.

• Since cold weather often triggers asthma, talk to the teacher or play group leader about the importance of being sure your child wears his coat, hat and mittens outside. These teachers have a multitude of shoes to tie and coats to zip, but it is important for your child not to be overlooked.

AGES SEVEN TO TWELVE

Most children who have asthma are diagnosed long before first grade even though asthma can occur in any person at any age. Most parents of elementary school children with asthma are very familiar with asthma's devastation and have worked many years to keep it under control.

As our children grow, we parents do too! We have become more accustomed to the changes we made when our little ones were born and have learned how to cope with things a little better. We have a better understanding of our children's early warning signals and triggers. Some of those may be subsiding while others become more pronounced. Some may disappear altogether or new allergens may just be surfacing.

What used to be "wheezing asthma" may now be "coughing asthma" or simply "seasonal hay fever."

When our children were little, we controlled their world as best as we could. We protected them, cradled them, wiped their noses, fed and diapered them. Now they have a life of their own. They go to school, to camp, play sports, climb trees and explore and grow more independent each day.

Our children are becoming young people with privileges and responsibilities. They get to spend the night at a friend's house, go on field trips and may even take a plane ride to visit Grandma and Grandpa. Certainly, if their asthma is well controlled, these great privileges become great memories. They also reward young people for accepting responsibility for their health.

Does your child know what to do to keep asthma under control when you are not around? Are you training your child to accept the responsibility to self-medicate according to your instruction? Are you teaching him warning signs that tell him he must get additional help? Are you teaching her to communicate effectively and calmly in the event that asthma does get out of control in a new situation?

The child in early elementary school years is very different from the early adolescent who is graduating from sixth grade. During these six years, he will experience both the rewards and consequences of life as he grows. He will test his limits and yours and mature before your very eyes. Watch carefully, he may even grow while you are looking!

You may already be at a point where asthma is well controlled. If your child's asthma required many hospitalizations, medications and your undivided attention for several years of her life, all that has probably changed by now. While it seems natural to you and me to adjust to controlled asthma, the transition may be more difficult for our children.

Children with chronic asthma have never known life without it. Their security is wrapped up in their disease.

When Brooke was nine, three years after asthma became well controlled, we discovered that she had many misconceptions of how life should be. I was not aware that my little princess would be confused by life with asthma under control. She'd grown up in a world where nurses and doctors focused individual attention on her physical and emotional needs on a regular basis and suddenly that attention was gone.

Brooke began to crave attention from teachers and other adults outside of our home. To receive the same amount of attention as her peers was not enough. Though having asthma and allergies had made her feel bad, there had always been someone there ready to wipe away the tears of her pain. Suddenly she was faced with the harsh realities of life and growing up without the comfort and protection of her illness.

Did we do something wrong by comforting her while she was sick? I don't believe so. Being sick was part of her life and pretending that it wasn't wouldn't have made her get well any faster. Even while Brooke's asthma was uncontrolled, she had family responsibilities and was disciplined. Our expressions of love to her were not dependent upon her being well or sick. We taught her to cooperate with her doctors and nurses and they could not have asked for a more loving, vibrant and energetic patient. However, controlled asthma reduced her contact with the people who were part of her sick life. Though she was well, she missed them and their affection.

S. R. Hirsch, M.D., an allergist in Milwaukee, Wisconsin, said it best in a recent letter to me: "It has been my impression after practicing allergy for twenty-five years that asthma is a very depressing disease, particularly for children. It means long hours spent taking medications, receiving injections, undergoing periodic episodes of ill-health, considerable discomfort and significant limitations in physical and scholastic activities. I think children need a clear-cut message of hope just as well as adults. I think they must understand that most children with asthma, if they follow the correct regimen, will be able to lead a perfectly normal life. I feel they must understand that their time for good health is not far off and that it is a goal that can be achieved."

Tools of the Trade

Your doctor may prescribe using a *nebulizer compressor* and a *flow meter*. Again, these are excellent tools for controlling and monitoring asthma. A *stethoscope* is also extremely helpful.

Nebulizer treatments may suddenly become a source of contention between you and your child. As elementary school kids become more aware of the world around them, they become self-conscious about doing anything that makes them feel different from their peers. Boys don't want to do it because it takes too much time and they don't want anyone to think they are wimpy. Girls don't like the treatments because they'd rather be doing something else. Younger children in this age group may enjoy working a puzzle, coloring, playing with clay or filling a sticker book during nebulizer treatments.

Discuss with your doctor the possibility of graduating to *spacer* treatments to substitute for one or two nebulizer treatments a day. The spacer gives your child the full benefit of the inhaled medication in a shorter period of time than the nebulizer. A spacer does not replace all the advantages of a nebulizer, but it can be helpful in motivating your child to take scheduled medications on time and in good spirits.

Medications

As your child grows older, it will become increasingly more challenging to coordinate scheduled medications with daily activities.

Talk to your child about the medications she takes. Help her understand the cause-and-effect relationship between medications and symptoms.

Some children have asthma only when they exercise. Consult with your doctor concerning a preexercise medication and a warm-up regimen.

Self-Management Skills

Your child is now getting old enough to assume responsibility for taking medications, telling you when medications are running low and having a working knowledge of triggers and early warning signals. These skills do not develop overnight. They must be taught one day at a time.

Even though children are capable of self-medicating, they may often forget whether they have taken their medication and actually skip a dose or take too much. When giving children the privilege of self-medicating, provide a chart and some stickers or stars so they can track their medication schedule. When you start letting your child self-medicate, become the supervisor. As he shows you he is capable, supervise from a distance. If there is ever a change in medications or dosage instructions, become the supervisor again.

Remind your child to use the inhaler properly if one has been prescribed. Even children who have been using them for years need to have their technique sharpened from time to time because they become a little cavalier about using them. Remember the correct procedure: the child should stand straight, take a deep breath, blow all his air out, put the inhaler in front of his mouth, depress the inhaler canister and immediately inhale slowly and deeply. If you notice medicine getting sprayed around your child's face, don't assume enough medication has gone into the lungs.

Seven- to twelve-year-olds can:

- Notify parent when medication is running low
- Record flow meter readings
- Self-medicate with age-appropriate supervision
- Recognize allergens, triggers and early warning signals
- Know what to do in case of an attack
- Know how to communicate effectively with teachers about their physical concerns
- Have a physical fitness plan that includes stamina-building activities
- Participate in most activities

Timely Tips

- Have your child bathe and wash and dry her hair before going to bed at night, especially during allergy season. Otherwise, allergens collected on the hair during the day are deposited on the pillowcase and the child wallows in it all night long. Be sure that the child's hair is thoroughly dry before tucking her in.

- A clean room, free of clutter and easy to dust, is still a must.

• Kids like to sleep overnight away from home with their friends once in a while. Many parents hesitate to let their children with asthma do this because they fear a possible attack during the middle of the night or burdening the host parents. Most of the time, everything will be just fine, but you must prepare your child and the host parents just in case. Then relax.

TEENS

The face of asthma management and pharmacology has changed so rapidly in recent years that many of today's teens grew up a couple of steps ahead of the improvements.

Many parents of teens with asthma are tired. They have exhausted the family budget looking for hope and help. They have submitted their children to testing, probing and counseling, and then repeated everything again. Their personal lives have suffered. They've done everything they can think of, and still they are left with a child who has chronic asthma and is missing out on life.

These parents are the most difficult for me to talk to because they have endured immeasurable pain and have no reward to show for it. Most of them do not care about new treatment plans or recent medical findings because they are too exhausted to invest their hope one more time. Many of these parents believe there really isn't anything new for asthmatics.

I realize there are exceptions to this broad general statement but who could blame a parent for fading after trying for over a decade to bring asthma under control. You know the roller coaster ride of emotions involved here. When our kids are healthy, things are very good. But when they are sick, things are very, very bad.

Not all adolescent asthmatics have uncontrolled asthma but by the time children are in their teens, they are either well controlled, managing to get by, or suffering. Chances are that if you are reading this book and you are the parent of a teenager with asthma, you probably have a child who is suffering.

Most books don't talk about teens who have asthma. It is almost as if they don't know how to reach them or that the authors think that most kids don't have asthma by the time they've reached adolescence. However, as this letter from a teen in Cornell, Wisconsin, indicates, asthma's impact on a teen's life is of major importance:

> *I am sixteen years old and I found out I had asthma for about three to four years now. I used to go to a doctor in Eau Claire but we stopped going to him about a year ago because he always seemed to put me on too much medication. My parents were worried about all the side effects. He always put me on prednisone. Once I was on it for a month and he never even saw me. It was prescribed over the phone!* WHAT ARE THE SIDE EFFECTS OF PREDNISONE?
>
> *Now I go to a different doctor. I was on 750 mg of theophylline a day.* WHAT ARE THE SIDE EFFECTS OF THEOPHYLLINE? *I was on four puffs in the morning and night of a steroid inhaler.* WHAT ARE THE SIDE EFFECTS OF A STEROID INHALER? *I was on two puffs morning and night of a Proventil inhaler.* WHAT ARE THE SIDE EFFECTS OF A PROVENTIL INHALER? *And now I am on an allergy pill morning and night called Trinalin Repetabs.*

WHAT ARE THE SIDE EFFECTS OF TRINALIN REPETABS? *Now I am slowly going off my medication. So far so good.*

I have lots of trouble telling when I am going to have an asthma attack. I usually don't know until I start wheezing. And my doctor said when you start wheezing it's too late. HOW ELSE CAN I TELL WHEN AN ASTHMA ATTACK IS GOING TO BE TRIGGERED?

I would like any other information on asthma you have available. THANKS AGAIN. ALSO, WHAT ARE MY CHANCES OF OUTGROWING ASTHMA? *I don't think they are good.*

The letter demonstrates a young woman's intense desire to understand her physical condition and to be a responsible partner in asthma management. She has asked many good questions that should have been answered long ago. Though the physical impact of her asthma is now being dealt with, this teenager's fears and concerns have not been relieved.

Sometimes we forget that our young people really do have the intellect to understand what is happening in their bodies. We forget that they care! I have every confidence that as this young woman pursues her goals in life, she will not be physically or emotionally handicapped by asthma. But there are many other teens who are already crippled because asthma has raged out of control all their lives and nothing appears to be stopping it.

I received a call one day from a school administrator regarding a sixteen-year-old boy who had asthma and missed an incredible amount of school. He noticed that when the boy did attend school, he seemed very depressed, lacked ambition and observed rather than participated. He said he talked to the boy and to his mother and he sensed that something was very wrong. He arranged for me to call the mother.

The mother said she had given up hope of her son ever "growing out of his asthma like the doctor said he would." She said that he refused to take his medicine because it made him feel sick. He was always wheezing, which tired him out so much that all he did was stay home and sleep. If he took his medicine, he became sick to his stomach, very irritable and difficult to manage. She just let him decide what he wanted to do.

I asked her if she talked to her doctor about these things and she said no, because "it never did any good talking to the doctor." He would just prescribe more medicine and it all made her son sick. I asked her when her son last visited the doctor and she said she thought it was about two years ago. She simply continues to refill his prescription whenever he runs out. That was not very often since he would only take the medicine if it was too hard to breathe.

Consider this child whose asthma has controlled his life for as long as he can remember. His father and his mother, upper middle class, educated parents, have accepted his asthma as their way of life. Unfortunately, they have also sentenced their son to a diminished existence.

When he is able to attend school, he doesn't know what is going on in any of his classes. He doesn't have any real friends. He is not a part of any clubs, sports activities or social groups. School is an important part of the adolescent's social development as well as educational training and he's missing it unnecessarily.

No one should be sentenced to a life of asthma out of control. More than ever, if your adolescent's asthma is still out of control, do not stop looking for a solution now. Those teens who have chronic, difficult to control (mild, moderate or severe) asthma, even if they are being treated by a very qualified doctor, may benefit from a second opinion. Sometimes a fresh point of view will provide the missing piece of the asthma management puzzle.

Tools of the Trade

When I responded to the Wisconsin sixteen-year-old's letter, I suggested that she obtain a peak flow meter and learn how to use it to help predict her asthma attacks before they start. A blow in the morning and a blow in the evening take only a few seconds, can be done in the privacy of her room and will provide her with the information she needs to initiate medication at the proper time. An attack prevented is insurance against embarrassment in front of peers and the side effects of medications.

Continue to use mite-proof mattress and pillow protectors.

Medications

Periodically, ask the doctor to observe your child's use of the inhaler.

Encourage your child to use the inhaler with confidence *before* he gets into wheezing situations *if a pretreatment plan has been prescribed.*

If your child is reluctant to take his medication, try to determine the reason. If your child resists using a medication that makes him feel sick, ask the doctor to adjust the current treatment plan or prescribe an alternative medication.

Self-Management Skills

Your child should have a very good understanding of the physiology of her asthma as well as a working knowledge of her asthma management plan. When you take a teen to the doctor, please avoid treating her as if she is only an object of discussion. Involve her in the decision-making processes. Encourage her to ask questions. Reassure her that her asthma may improve as she gets older but it is important to control it *now*.

Kids with low self-esteem will need more encouragement as they learn asthma self-management techniques. Praise your child's strengths and try to uncover fears. For example, he may avoid dating for fear of having an asthma attack or he may believe that his asthma is contagious. Help him plan a strategy for avoiding allergens and premedicating before going on a date. Remind him that asthma is not contagious and to go ahead and kiss his date if she doesn't mind. Your child will appreciate your willingness to see things from his perspective.

Many teens who have asthma lead very active, normal lives. Your child may not be athletically inclined but he should be able to participate in physically challenging activities at a reasonable level. The key word here is participate. It should be obvious to others that your child has an "I'll try" attitude. If he is unable to participate in physical activities after following the doctor's treatment plan, a reevaluation is in order. If necessary, ask the doctor to develop a physical fitness plan that will increase lung capacity at a very gradual rate. By the way, if your teen can boogie at the sock hop, he can hustle on the gym floor as well!

If your son or daughter accepts responsibility for his or her

asthma management, reward your child with the independence sought. You could help your teen find part-time employment. Maybe you could help him study to obtain a driv-
er's permit. Encourage your teen to have friends visit in your
home and allow him *reasonable* freedom to visit others at
their homes. Show your teen that appropriate behavior yields
not only better health but greater personal freedom.

As children get older, they become a more active part of
the decision-making process. They learn to listen to their
bodies, to know when to slow down or to push themselves.
They become less dependent upon Mom and Dad and more
confident of their own ability to handle their asthma. Teach
them how to tell if their inhaled medication is running low,
how to take and record their own peak flow meter readings.
Teach them to take steps to control their environment and
make up missed schoolwork. Encourage them as they assume responsibility for these things.

There will be many decisions to make as children grow up
with asthma. You should define those areas for which your
child will be responsible and those areas that will remain
your responsibility. Though you and your teen will work together to get and keep asthma controlled, you will probably
be the one who is ultimately responsible for making sure the
plan is followed until the day your child leaves home.

Timely Tips

- Inhalers are often awkward to carry, especially for young
  men who don't carry purses and want to look cool. Few
  teens have the confidence to establish their own standard
  of cool. Even so, it helps to have a couple of extra inhalers
  around. One should be kept in his three-ring binder (in a
  clear plastic zippered pencil case) to accompany him to his

classes and one in the school nurse's office. Girls should keep their inhalers handy in their purses at all times. Some schools do not permit children to carry inhalers, largely due to fears about their use and their legal responsibilities. However, these fears are unfounded and compound problems for the children who need them. Discuss this with the school.

- Allergies are not cool either. My oldest son, Mike, has seasonal hay fever. Until 1987, he suffered greatly for about three weeks in the spring and six weeks in the summer and fall. The allergies made his eyes swell and weep and his nose run. More often than not, his teachers would send him to the clinic suspecting pinkeye. If I gave him the prescribed antihistamines, he would fall asleep in class or his friends would tease him about "using drugs."

  Mike was good-natured about the ribbing, but he was missing too much school. I called his allergist and she prescribed a regimen of three nose sprays, eye drops and a nonsedating antihistamine. After he got the current allergy flare under control, he could discontinue two of the nasal sprays and use the remaining one to prevent future problems. Three weeks before the next allergy season, we started the preventive part of his allergy control plan and it worked like a charm.

- Teens like lots of clutter in their rooms, lots of things that are huge no-no's on the environmental control list your doctor gave you. This is one area where parents must tread carefully. Sit down with your child and explain the reasoning behind keeping the sleeping quarters free of allergens, then ask your child to show you which possessions he feels must stay in the room and which he would be willing to keep in a storage closet outside the room.

LETTING GO

It was a normal Saturday except that Michael's peak flow readings were dropping. We're still not sure what happened, whether it was a heralding of the chicken pox which followed the next day or if he ate something which he was allergic to, but whatever happened, it happened fast and when Michael stood up and said, "It's hard to breathe, Mom, and my nebulizer treatment is not working," I knew we were in trouble.

A quick assessment with his peak flow meter told me that Michael was in serious condition. A flood of fear overwhelmed me as I watched the color leave his face. Numbly, I dialed 911 and called for the Rescue Unit. Shaking, I fumbled to get the cap off the Epi-pen, the shot of adrenaline that the doctor prescribed for emergencies. If ever there was an emergency, this was it.

Outwardly, I was calm because I didn't want to frighten Michael, but inwardly, I was scared to death. He began to turn blue around his lips, so I looked out the window to see if any help was on the way and saw that the Rescue Unit had gone to the wrong house. I ran outside and yelled, "Over here."

Within minutes Michael was hooked up and "wired for sound." The barrage of questions followed . . . one paramedic asking about possible causes and the other adapting the treatment. I watched them working as a team with the doctor (who was located at the hospital emergency room), and knew he would be all right when I heard the words, "I am getting a hiss going through," meaning Michael was beginning to move air again.

Already I was thinking ahead to what I would never give him to eat again. Then I thought about never letting him out of my sight again. Then I realized how foolish I would look with a seven-year-old skateboarder attached to me. I was going to draw the line at skydiving and honeymoons, but an hour after recovering from this frightening episode, a very normal Michael wanted to go outside to play. Taking a deep breath, I said yes.

Michael is your normal everyday boy who collects bugs, gushes their guts, rides bikes, skateboards, draws dinosaurs and periodically drives his parents crazy. He just has asthma and some very severe reactions to certain foods.

Every day parents practice letting go of their children without even noticing. It is scarier for parents of children with asthma to let go. However, let go we must or we *may find ourselves skateboarding and sky-diving beyond our years.*   *—Janice Berger, a mother in Reston, Virginia*

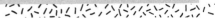

Your child should then be responsible for thorough weekly cleanings in return for the privilege of keeping the possessions. If your child cannot keep up with the dust and clutter in his room, he loses the privilege of keeping his possessions the way he wants.

• Unfortunately, our children have been sold a very self-destructive bill of goods throughout their formative years. Television, movies, certain rock music, etc. have led young people to assume that they can safely dabble in drugs, alcohol and sex without consequence. However, the physical consequences are far greater for our children. Drugs and alcohol compromise their bodies further and if a person has an asthma attack under the influence of either, it is unlikely he or she will be able to respond properly. Sexual exploration may lead to pregnancy, venereal disease or AIDS. Educate your children. Help them understand the reality of the consequences.

AT EVERY AGE

A great deal of the success our children will have in managing their illness will depend on how early in life the asthma is brought under control and how consistent we as parents are in teaching them to manage the asthma.

To achieve control of asthma, there must be a plan. If your

children do not understand their involvement in the plan, they become the object of our manipulation. Through learning asthma self-management skills, they learn skills needed for living.

From the very beginning, you must discipline your child with unsavory consequences for inappropriate actions. If your efforts to discipline are floundering, you may want to seek advice from a counselor, pastor or psychologist. Ask for help in establishing the boundaries, creative means for encouraging and setting family goals. Sometimes all it takes is a reaffirmation of who's in charge to bridge the "communication gap."

Our children with asthma, even more so than children without asthma, must learn how to plan ahead, respond in an emergency, be reliable and consistent and stand alone. After all, they won't always have Mom and Dad to be thinking for them.

If asthma continues to be so difficult to control that your child is constantly in and out of the hospital and unable to attend school, medical consultation at an intensive asthma facility is in order.

CHAPTER 9

ASTHMA
GOES TO
SCHOOL

ASTHMA IS NOT A PROBLEM KEPT QUIETLY AT home. Attacks can occur anywhere, and our kids need to be prepared to handle them wherever they are, including school. At the same time, we have to prepare teachers and school administrators to help if an attack happens.

YOUR CHILD'S TEACHER

Most teachers will have encountered children with asthma before your child entered the school. Your job is to learn how much they know about asthma, make them aware of the many misconceptions that can affect a child's developing self-image and describe the individual characteristics of (and the management plan for) your child's asthma.

Before school starts, call the school requesting any forms that may be required for children using medications at school. Try to have these forms completed before you meet with the principal, school nurse and the child's teacher.

It is nice to have both parents at the initial meeting. It lets the school know that both parents care. And what one parent may forget, the other one will most likely remember.

Approach the meeting willing to learn as well as willing to inform. In fact, a good way to open the meeting is to acknowledge that this is your first time sending an asthmatic child to school and that you realize the school has encountered kids with asthma many times in the past. Then remember what you came to this meeting to do: to introduce your child and the unique characteristics of his asthma to a school that may not know him at all. Here are some matters to discuss:

- Stress that asthma is not contagious and is not a psychological disease.

- Discuss the difference between an attack and wheezing while on medications, and the symptoms that require parental or medical attention.

- Explain that triggers must be respected and avoided. Provide a list of triggers for each educator present. These could include class pets, foods, chalk dust, plants, pollens, fumes from chemicals used in science projects, school construction dust, paint fumes, exercise, barometric or temperature changes and season changes, to name just a few. It will be particularly helpful for teachers planning class parties and "ice cream treat days" to be aware that certain foods will cause problems.

- Demonstrate the use of the inhaler, peak flow meter, spacer or nebulizer. Make sure you leave a spare inhaler or two at the school and accept responsibility for replacing them before they are empty.

- Provide a flow meter and make sure your child and teacher know how to use it. Have the appropriate and inappropriate range numbers taped on the meter.

- Make sure the teachers know the difference between medications (especially inhaled medications) similar in shape or appearance (such as Proventil and Intal, Proventil being used to control wheezing and Intal to prevent an attack due to an inhaled trigger).

- Make sure medication is labeled properly and directions for use are updated as your doctor's instructions change.

- Discuss the possible side effects of the drugs. Remember that side effects are often signs that the medications must be adjusted and that the asthma is not optimally under control.

- Remind the teacher to remain calm during an attack and to encourage other children who might be present to remain calm, too. Your child should already be aware of the value of remaining calm. Usually, a person needing help will communicate that need aggressively. The person with asthma shouldn't, because getting excited can make matters worse. Since help often comes at the same rate of intensity as it is requested, teachers might underestimate the seriousness of an attack if they don't know this.

- Discuss any physical limitations the child may have and develop an alternate plan for physical activity and development if necessary.

- It is best to have a specific procedure neatly typed explaining what to do in case of an attack as well as on days that I call "yellow alert"—when symptoms require medications and a watchful eye—because things could go well or not so well. Always have an alternative plan of action in writing in case you cannot be reached. Provide separate copies for the school nurse and teacher.

- If your child has a history of sudden-onset asthma or reactions to foods, bee stings, etc., provide a small card with his picture at the top and a concise description of the problem and how to treat it in bold letters. This should be kept in plain view in the school nurse's office so that your child will be rapidly identified and attended to, even if the clinic is being staffed by a volunteer or someone else who may not know him.

- Work with the teacher to establish a system for getting make-up assignments. Whether you pick them up yourself, get them over the telephone or have the teacher send them home with another child, there should be a plan for helping your child keep up in spite of missed school days.

- Many schools do not have the services of a school nurse. These schools rely on volunteer help. However, as medical science enables a greater number of our physically challenged kids to go to school, I believe it is even more important for the schools to be prepared to meet the medical challenge by staffing with school nurses. If there is no school nurse at your school, contact your local school board to find out how your school can get one.

Above all, before you leave the meeting, confirm that your objective is to keep the number of absences to a minimum and the exposure to a positive-learning environment to a maximum. Don't forget to balance the seriousness of asthma with the positive effect of responsible management. Managing asthma will most certainly develop character and self-discipline.

GETTING READY TO START SCHOOL

When talking to your young child about starting school for the first time, appeal to his sense of adventure and curiosity. Look for opportunities to introduce your child to handling an attack when you are not present. At this age, kids are more inclined to tell you what's on their minds if they are rolling clay or coloring at the kitchen table. This is a perfect time to pick up a crayon and start talking to your child. "What would you do?" games spark imagination and reveal a lot more than you'd guess. "What would you do if you were the captain of a ship and you saw a little boy having an asthma attack?" The "what would you do" questions eventually lead to, "if you were the teacher and a little boy had an attack on the playground" and then "what do you think you will do if you have a hard time breathing at school?" Don't forget to praise thoughtful and correct answers.

ALLERGIES AT SCHOOL

Children who suffer from allergy symptoms with or without asthma often have a difficult time managing at school. Fortunately, most allergies to airborne pollutants (such as pollen) are seasonal. But some children experience allergy symptoms throughout the school year. The most common outward appearance of a child troubled by allergies is red, itchy, swollen and watery eyes, accompanied by stuffy head and nose. Sometimes the eyes are so swollen, red and itchy that the condition is mistaken for conjunctivitis (pinkeye).

Medications traditionally prescribed to combat the al-

A SOLO VIGIL

Matthew started first grade today. He started in a brand-new school completely carpeted with 100 percent nylon plastic and adhered with Armstrong's #10 adhesive . . . it looks great but for the first time since early summer, Matthew's peak flow meter readings would not reach normal. The odor triggered the problem and I'm afraid we are in for a long night. The extra meds have been given and now the long night's vigil begins. As usual, it will be a solo vigil because my husband is on a business trip . . . Support system? I haven't any. We live in rural Virginia where asthma is considered as serious as a hangnail. To compound matters, the hospital is twenty-one miles away.—Mother in Powhatan, Virginia

lergy often lull your child to sleep in the classroom. Nonallergic children are sometimes alarmed by the altered appearance of their classmate and (especially in seventh through twelfth grades) chide the allergic student about being a "druggie." Recently, new medications have been released that do not cause sleepiness or hyperactivity. Terfenadine (seldane) is a drug used to relieve symptoms once they have begun, also without sleepiness or that spacey feeling for most users. Others in this category include claritin and hisminol.

Cromolyn sodium (Intal, Nasalcrom Opticrom), when used before and during allergy season, has produced excellent results in preventing allergy symptoms without the side effects commonly associated with antihistamines.

In addition to taking medications, allergy patients often find relief if they rinse their face frequently during the day and avoid outdoor activities during high pollen or mold spore counts and dry, windy days.

PHYSICAL EDUCATION

"**A**sthmatics should not be expected to participate in physical education" is as dangerous a myth as "children grow out of their asthma." Kids with asthma *can* and should participate in P.E.; however, many children need a prescribed plan for reaching fitness goals. The physical education classes required in most schools can be a good place for your child to explore her limits and build stamina to help reach new levels of conditioning.

Parents should meet with their child's physical education teacher before the school year begins. Provide a list of triggers and early warning signals and what to do if the child has a sudden attack in class. Provide a peak flow meter and show the teacher how it is used. Explain that flow meter readings in the green zone mean that the child should be expected to participate in class to his best ability, yellow zone readings mean if the child exercises, it should be a low-level activity that is preceded by prescribed medications (a note or phone call to the home should follow). If the child's flow meter readings are in the red zone, an indication of crisis, he doesn't belong at school.

A flow meter can also be a useful visual aid for the child who believes he or she really can't participate in sports. If the peak flow meter reading is normal and no wheezing is present, gentle encouragement to premedicate and participate (even if at a low level) will open up doors of freedom for children who live in fear of impending attacks. The peak flow meter can then be used to demonstrate lung capacity before and after exercise. Building lung capacity is important for asthmatics but also difficult if there is fear of an exercise-induced attack.

You may have to ask the teacher to excuse your child from participating in outdoor activities when the pollen count is exceedingly high or on cold, blustery days. Help the teacher understand that he or she should not base expectations of how your child can perform on their experience with other children who have asthma.

There is rarely an excuse for a child with asthma to sit idle during physical education classes just as there is rarely an excuse for him to be pushed beyond what he can do. For children in need of a physical education program geared toward people with asthma, there is an exercise video that can be used by the P.E. teacher or in the privacy of your home. It is called *Aerobics for Asthmatics.* Nancy Hogshead, a 1984 Olympic Gold Medalist (who also has asthma), along with Kathy Lampl, M.D., and Stanley Wolf, M.D., designed this inspirational, educational and physically challenging forty-five-minute exercise routine for people with asthma.

Dusty gyms are a serious problem for many children with asthma and allergies. I've seen large globs of dust swirling in the air of elementary school gyms. That alone is enough to make eyes water, noses itch, and can also trigger asthma. Since asthma and allergies account for the largest number of days that children are absent each year, it is reasonable to expect that the gym floor be mopped each night. In many schools, the children are not permitted to wear dark-soled shoes or shoes with deep ridges while in P.E. because it makes it more difficult to keep the floor clean. The dust and dirt that would scar the floor also irritate the airways of those children who have asthma and allergies.

Your child's physical education teacher is less likely to make the mistake of pushing your child too far if you provide specific guidelines. Do not ask her to be your child's caretaker. Just ask her to be aware and considerate of your child's health. Let the teacher know that what she does at school is likely to affect life at home later in the evening. Do not make demands of any teacher even if in your opinion she is wrong. Be a creative communicator. Be an advocate for your child according to the policies of the school. There is always another avenue for appeal if your case warrants it.

SHOULD MY CHILD STAY HOME TODAY?

It is often difficult to determine if your child should stay home from school when asthma is a problem. Good communication between teacher, parent and child will enable the child to attend school on those marginal days when you wonder if the child would be any worse off at school than at home. The following guidelines are suggested by the Center for Interdisciplinary Research on Immunologic Diseases at Georgetown University, Washington, D.C., in their publication *You Can Control Asthma:*

Your child can go to school with:

- a stuffy nose, but no wheezing
- mild wheezing that clears after giving medicine
- the ability to do his usual daily activities
- no difficulty breathing

Keep your child home with:

- evidence of infection, sore throat or swollen, painful neck glands
- a fever over 100 degrees F. orally; face hot and flushed
- wheezing that continues to be labored one hour after medicine is given
- weakness or tiredness that makes it hard to take part in usual daily activities
- difficulty breathing

The reading on your child's peak flow meter can also help you decide. A lower than normal reading, coupled with other early warning signals (such as a chronic cough, pale skin color, etc.) may be a warning that an asthma attack is nearing. Parents should medicate their children as instructed by the doctor, watch for appropriate responses and base the decision to send the child to school on the child's response to the medications. If the child is sent to school, please notify the teacher that your child is in preasthma stages but controlled with medications. If possible or indicated, go up to the school to check on your child just before the next medication is due. A quick assessment with the flow meter and listening to the child's chest will tell you what you need to know.

Some children's asthma is worse in the morning than midday. This can be a problem with morning kindergarten or preschool programs. Try to arrange for afternoon schooling for the younger children as this tendency may improve as the child gets older. Older children with this same problem need not miss an entire day of school.

THE EFFECT OF THEOPHYLLINE ON LEARNING AND SCHOOL BEHAVIOR

Concern over the effect of one asthma medication, theophylline, on learning and behavior has been raised in recent years, not only by parents but the medical community as well. Much of what has been published in news reports is misleading and alarming when a balanced presentation of the information would be far more beneficial.

Reports that theophylline *causes* learning disabilities or attention-deficit disorders are simply unfounded; however, the side effects of this bronchodilating medication can *mimic* clinical behavior and learning problems in some children.

The researchers estimated that the caffeine in three cups of coffee has about the same bronchodilating effect of a standard dose of theophylline. Three cups of coffee would make most of us feel and act differently if we were not used to drinking it.

Some children become excitable, find it difficult to concentrate, are easily irritated or have trouble getting along with others when taking theophylline. They sometimes have trouble assimilating abstract information that requires a motor response such as writing the equation for a mathematical word problem or following a series of commands. These are also some of the hallmarks of learning and behavior problems. If theophylline is the culprit of a child's behavior problems, the symptoms should disappear after the medication is discontinued and return if restarted.

Not all children taking theophylline will have these side effects. Parents may not be aware that their child has a problem at school until his behavior or academic performance has established a pattern that qualifies the child for testing. Teachers may not know that the child is taking a medication that can, in some children, give the appearance of learning or behavior problems.

Children with asthma may also have a genuine learning problem not associated with their medication. They can have behavior disorders that have nothing to do with theophylline. However, if a teacher suspects a learning or behavior problem exists, and your child is taking theophylline, don't panic. Ask your doctor to help you and the child's teacher determine whether the theophylline is indeed causing your child to appear as though he has learning or behavior problems.

If you suspect a problem it will be helpful to keep a daily diary which tracks symptoms, medications (sometimes the combined effects of taking multiple medications necessary to halt an attack can compound the problem), peak flow meter readings and behaviors. *The Asthma Organizer,* by Debbie Scherrer, Martha Vetter White, M.D., and me has a daily diary which could serve this purpose. See the Resources section.

In a September 1986 report on theophylline, Dr. Stanley Szefler, National Jewish Center for Immunology and Respiratory Medicine, addresses the subject of adverse effects including school behavior problems:

"There are several well-described undesirable effects attributed to theophylline including gastrointestinal distress, seizures and cardiac arrhythmias. Of recent concern is the recognition of potential effects of theophylline on learning and behavior in children. Several studies recognized an increased incidence of adverse effects, such as nausea and nervousness, with theophylline therapy in comparisons to cromolyn. These usually occurred in the first five weeks of therapy. Parents also identified school behavior problems.

"These observations precipitated a follow-up study by Furakawa et al. in a selected group of children whose parents expressed concern about learning or behavior difficulties. The children first received psychological testing during theophylline therapy and were re-evaluated after crossing over to cromolyn. The investigators concluded that the children were less restless, distractible and irritable; also, they were more manageable and slept better during the second observation period as noted by the mothers of these children. Psychological testing determined that improvements in attention, concentration and/or memory were observed in the second study period. Limitations in this study included the small sample size, selection process for study patients, absence of a control group, potential for recognized improvement as influenced by practice and the parents' expectations.

Nevertheless, these observations require careful consideration and identify the need for further studies." And more investigations are currently under way.

But as Dr. Szefler also noted, "There is no doubt that theophylline is an effective bronchodilator for the treatment of acute and chronic respiratory distress . . ." and has its place in the asthma management plan.

The question is, based on the amount of knowledge we have concerning a specific medication, how can it or should it be used to meet the physical needs of my child? Asthma therapies are changing rapidly as technology provides more alternatives and information. Applying that information to your child's needs is a decision for both you and your informed doctor to make. Just don't forget to inform your child's teachers.

BE A VOLUNTEER

There is probably no better way to get a realistic picture of your child's school life than to be a volunteer. As volunteers, parents demonstrate their willingness to serve and communicate productively. As volunteers, parents become visible, accessible participants in the educational process of their children. Parental presence in the school can provide a sense of security for younger children and it gives parents the opportunity to casually check the child periodically. Probably even more important is the sense of security parents of asthmatic children feel when they become involved.

One mother of a child with asthma volunteers in the school clinic one day a week. Another mother volunteers as a reading teacher, kindergarten workshop mother, computer re-source helper and library helper, all in four hours one day a week. Other parents assist with cafeteria duty, or are active in the PTA. Some volunteers are employed outside of their homes and others are not. Some have small children in tow while others form babysitting co-ops with other mothers of wee ones.

The more visible a parent is, the more likely a teacher is to mention something that may seem too trivial to require a phone call. On those days when the child's asthma is mar-ginal, it is easier to send a child to school when the parent will be nearby.

Volunteering at school is great fun, too. It requires plan-ning and can sometimes be inconvenient, but the rewards are great and the new friends are many, something that parents with asthmatic children need an extra dose of!

MAKING UP IS NOT SO HARD TO DO

Making up missed schoolwork is not as hard to do if asthma is under control. The occasional flares that keep a child from school should not keep a child behind in school-work. Parents and teachers should work out ahead of time a system of collecting assignments and assisting children when they miss school. In a study by Robert Strunk, M.D., children who missed up to a quarter of the school year were able to stay on grade level when classroom assignments were com-pleted at home.

Making up missed schoolwork can be very difficult when asthma is out of control, especially if there are learning difficulties, problems with self-esteem or social problems. However difficult and distressing the situation may be, *parents and teachers must address this problem completely if the child is to be taught to lead a productive life.*

First, get the asthma under control. Chronic absenteeism is not acceptable and indicates poorly controlled asthma. Most children with controlled asthma can attend school with very few asthma-related absences.

If the medications are not controlling the asthma, talk to the doctor about readjustments. If things are not going well at school, take another look at your home. Make sure your home is free of known allergens. Read books and literature about responsible asthma management. Be a participant in your child's health care plan. Do not be afraid of getting a second opinion if you need confirmation of the decisions you make with your doctor—but get asthma under control. Then address psychological, social or learning difficulties until the problems are resolved.

Children with asthma out of control often become discouraged with trying to cope with their illness at school, especially as they grow older. They feel different, embarrassed and physically tired. Homebound instruction is available in many states for children with chronic illness; however, few children who have asthma require this service on a permanent basis. Unlike the classroom setting, home instruction (for the sake of accommodating asthma) cannot provide a child with the kind of social interaction with peers that is so vital to normal social development. But homebound instruction can be very helpful on a temporary basis.

CHAPTER 10

SPORTS AND OUTDOOR ADVENTURES

M ANY OF US HAVE FOND CHILDHOOD MEMO-
ries of camping in the "wilderness" with our family or
friends, earning merit badges in Scouts, going off to summer
camp or playing a team sport. Though the activities were always fun, there was an element of learning, exploring and
growing that we can appreciate now that we're parents ourselves.

It is in camping, Scouts, and sporting activities that our

children can develop confidence, build relationships, compete, and investigate their personal and physical limitations outside our direct supervision and protection. They may even outdistance our expectations.

SPORTS

Exercise is good for everyone! It is a myth that people with asthma cannot exercise. People with asthma just do it a little differently. A preexercise medication plan may be helpful if prescribed, however. Some people avoid problems by warming up and gradually increasing their exercise level and maintaining that level before gradually cooling down. Some children and adults must do a combination of both, but most find they can then participate in the activity of their choosing without limitation.

It has been long established that exercise strengthens the cardiovascular system, builds muscle tone and improves general health. Exercise does not cure asthma. But the more physically fit a person, the more likely he is to be healthy and to require less medication. This is true for most chronic illnesses, including heart ailments, diabetes and even arthritis.

Organized sports offer great opportunities for children to explore their physical limits. Children with controlled asthma are more likely to have a successful experience than those children whose asthma is constantly defeating them. Controlled asthma allows children to compete and play among their peers. Children with uncontrolled asthma who have the determination to compete, do so *in spite* of suffering with asthma.

Some very fine athletes have asthma. One such young man from Rockville, Maryland, said he felt his asthma made him a better competitor. He learned the meaning of persevering, keeping sight of his goal and working hard to reach it.

And if you think that children with asthma can not "go for the gold," in 1984, approximately 10 percent of the U.S. Olympic athletes were diagnosed as having exercise-induced asthma. Of the sixty-six athletes on the team with a positive diagnosis, forty-one went on to win medals.

With three boys who love sports in our family, Brooke was not about to be left out. She plays basketball and likes to golf, has taken gymnastics and loves to swim. She participates energetically in each of these sports. However, she must prepare her body before each activity, except for swimming, because one of Brooke's asthma triggers is exercise.

Depending on her peak flow meter readings, the preparation may be as simple as using her albuterol inhaler (Ventolin, Proventil) twenty minutes before activity. Other times she will have to add her cromolyn sodium (Intal) inhaler. Brooke is also on daily medications, none of which cause any side effects. She knows how to prevent an asthma attack and what to do if one should start "squeezing her chest."

If there is any deviation from her prevention plan, Brooke will have an asthma attack in the middle of her activity. For example, in the winter of 1987, when she was the only girl on her basketball team, she forgot to bring her inhaler to one of the games. It was also one of the few times I did not have an extra inhaler in my purse. Brooke played the second quarter of the game, racing up and down the court with her cheeks flushed and braids trailing. The first half ended and the team huddled around the coach for the game plan for the second half. Then I noticed that Brooke was not in the huddle. When

I looked for her, I found her hidden in a recessed doorway in the gym breathing slowly and deeply and fumbling for her inhaler in her coat pockets.

"Are you having trouble breathing, Brooke?" I asked, in spite of the obvious.

"No," she fibbed. "I'll be okay in a minute. I'm just wheezing a little."

I sat on the floor next to her and helped her look for her inhaler. The second half started. The coach asked her if she was going to be able to play. "The fourth quarter," she said. "I'll be okay by the fourth quarter."

But within a few minutes, Brooke said, "I can't do it anymore. I better get home and get a breathing treatment, Mommy."

By sitting next to Brooke, I was aware that the controlled breathing exercises were very labored and what Brooke really needed was her medication, but giving her a few minutes' time allowed her to make a decision (one which I would have made if she hadn't) and also helped her realize that she must always be responsible about carrying her inhaler. Though it was a difficult lesson for her to learn, the tearful disappointment of missing the second half of the game taught her to be prepared in the future.

Also, Brooke understands that her asthma attack was not only exercise-induced but compounded by allergens in the gym. Brooke's basketball practices and games are usually held in elementary school gyms, two of which are extremely dusty. Big clumps of dust swirl through the air each time a player dribbles the ball down the sides of the court. Brooke's face will become splotchy, her nose and eyes will become itchy and she will start to wheeze if we do not treat her with preventive medications before she plays.

This year, Brooke was on a basketball team with another

child, Greg, who has asthma. His mother was suspicious that exercise might be a trigger because he looked as if he was "running tired." His mouth was wide open and he seemed to lag behind the rest of the children on the team even though they were smaller than he. She took a peak flow meter reading before the next practice and then, when she noticed him running tired, discreetly took another peak flow meter reading. His reading was very low, so she had him use his inhaler, which helped. She took another peak flow meter reading after basketball practice and he had improved but was still not in his green or healthy zone. One hour later, his peak flow readings were normal. His mother later called the doctor, who confirmed her suspicions and gave her a pretreatment plan to follow until the next appointment.

Children and adults can be tested for exercise-induced asthma with pulmonary function testing before, during and after exercise but *most* parents notice symptoms well enough that the only purpose served in testing is to confirm that which is already observable. A simpler version of that test is to use the peak flow meter in the same way that Greg's mom did.

Exercise-induced asthma does not always make a patient wheeze. It can cause the sufferer to cough, choke and gag, too! Sometimes, the patient even vomits following exercise. Many times exercise-induced asthma is first experienced following a bout with bronchitis or pneumonia, a time when the lungs are not quite healed from infection.

Here are some exercise tips:

- For children who play outdoor sports who will encounter dust, wind, grass, pollens and temperature changes— where there's a will, there's a play. Remind your child to use preventive medications according to your doctor's instructions. These can include nasal sprays, eye drops, inhalers and nonsedating antihistamines.

- Children who participate in winter indoor sports should wear warm clothing to and from the gym. Don't allow a sweating, heated child to run out into cold weather even if it is only a short sprint to the car. The older the child, the more likely he will try to do this. If your son or daughter doesn't want to be reminded to dress properly in front of friends, warn him or her ahead of time not to forget!

- Swimming is a great sport, especially for children with asthma. There is little loss of body fluids, and allergens are not a problem (except for a few children who get hives or asthma from cold water). In colder climates, private and public indoor swim facilities allow children to participate year round.

- Talk to the coach about your child's asthma. Tell the coach that your child wants to play and has the ability to contribute to the team. Reassure the coach that you do not hold him responsible for ensuring that your child uses medications but that he needs to be aware of signs to watch for and know when to pull your child off the playing court or field. Provide the coach with emergency information. In communicating this information, be sensitive that it may cause him concern or even be frightening. Stick to the facts, leave out any horror stories and tell the coach there is no need to keep your child on the bench. Whatever you do, don't keep your child's coach in the dark about handling your child's asthma!

- If needed, take the portable nebulizer with you to your child's sporting activities. However, don't call attention to your child's asthma by carting it around in an obvious manner. Most attacks which are triggered by exercise will subside quickly after a couple of puffs of an inhaler followed by controlled diaphragmatic breathing. Many times, the child recovers sufficiently to be back in the action in ten or fifteen minutes.

• Be certain that your child keeps adequately hydrated.

• Don't be afraid to bring the flow meter to games. If you suspect a problem, take your child aside in private, take a reading, assess and then respond appropriately to your child's need. As your child gets older, parents need to be less visible with asthma tools. The less attention drawn to the child having an attack the better.

CAMP MINI-WHEEZE-NO-MORE

Choose your child's summer camp carefully. If it is your child's first camp experience, I would recommend an asthma camp (see Resources section). We've received letters from parents all over the country who were thrilled with the many wonderful activities and self-management skills their children learned while away. Not only do the children have fun, but they meet other children who require breathing treatments and take allergy shots.

If you can answer yes to most of these questions, chances are your child is ready for camp:

• Is the child able to make new friends?

• Is the child eager to stay at a friend's house overnight?

- Has the child overcome his fear of the dark?

- Has the child had any previous day camp or overnight camping experiences?

- Has the child been involved in any peer group activities, such as Scouting?

- Has the child had opportunities to be independent? Does he help with chores or shop by himself for small items?

- Does the child relate well to adults?

- Does the child relate well to groups of children?

- Is the child friendly and outgoing?

- Is the child inquisitive and eager to share newly learned information?

- Is the child responsible for his own personal hygiene; that is, can he dress alone and bathe himself?

—From Merle S. Scherr, M.D., cofounder of the Former Camp Bronco Junction, West Virginia

Some of the asthma camps have a certain number of openings for those who cannot afford to pay. Check with your local Asthma and Allergy Foundation chapter, American Lung Association, the Lung Line, the American Academy of Allergy & Immunology or the American College of Allergy & Immunology for their camp listings.

Regardless of your choice of camps, asthma or regular, pay strict attention to sleeping quarters, staffing, medical personnel, location of nearest emergency room and food. Will your child have phone privileges? Will you be able to call the camp to check on your child's health and to ease your mind if necessary?

It is always nice if you can find a camp which has air-conditioned sleeping quarters but this may be hard to find. Within reason, dorms should be kept clean and free of dust and should not have a musty, mildewy smell. Parents are often asked to supply sheets, pillows, and other bedding for their own child.

Bring or send your own mite- and allergen-proof mattress and pillow encasing for your child's bedding. To avoid other children misinterpreting your gesture as an indication that your child wets the bed, arrive early or use (or send with your child) a polyester cotton/vinyl encasing that looks and feels like anything but plastic.

Many times, generous doctors and nurses will volunteer their services at asthma camps. Those I have spoken to enjoy the experience so much, they return with their families year after year.

Children with asthma attending a regular summer camp will probably not have the advantage of an asthma specialist on staff. Many times, the counselors are inadequately prepared to make timely decisions concerning a wheezing child and may wait until too late to get help. They have so many children to care for that your requests may seem unreasonable. However, if the camp is willing to help, provide a written list of allergens, early warning signals and demonstrate the use and administration of medications.

As most camps are located in remote areas, medical help can be distant. Parents should find out where their child would be taken in an emergency. If the camp doctor thinks that asthma is a psychological problem, or the emergency facility is more than thirty minutes away, it is probably not wise to register your child at that camp.

If food allergies are a serious problem, pack your child's special foods with simple directions for preparation and leave them with the manager of the "chow hall." Check the camp menu for hidden food allergy problems, i.e., chili thickened with peanut butter or green beans cooked with butter.

We have all heard horror stories about camp emergencies. However, most asthma problems, even those at camp, can be avoided with careful planning.

FAMILY CAMPING

Before you go camping, pitch the tent outside on a warm sunny day to air musty odors. Tumble sleeping bags in the drier to remove pollens and kill mold spores. If the sleeping bags smell musty, machine wash or have them dry cleaned. After each trip, wash and dry the sleeping bags and store them in plastic garbage bags before putting them away. That way, they will be ready for the next camping trip.

Place the sleeping bag on a camp cot or on an air mattress that is laid on top of a sheet of plastic. Avoid down or wool sleeping bags as they tend to irritate allergies in some children.

Tent camping is fun but so is camping in a motor home or travel trailer. This type of camping provides many of the luxuries of home and is easier to keep allergen-free than tent camping.

Poison ivy, poison oak and poison sumac rashes can be irritating to any child, but especially so for the child with asthma and allergies. Teach a class in poison plant identification at the start of the camping trip!

Camping is fun but finding medical help in an emergency is not. Locate the emergency room upon arrival at the campsite. Chances are that if you will need it, it will be during the night, so look for landmarks that will help you remember your way. Do not isolate your family in remote areas without some way of obtaining help within thirty minutes.

If a nebulizer has been prescribed, a portable unit suitable for outdoor use is a must for campers with asthma. A portable nebulizer will give your family the freedom to take a hike to a waterfall, go for a bike ride or swim at the lake all afternoon. You may never need it, but if you do, it is there and the family outing is uninterrupted. The peace of mind it provides is worth borrowing, renting or purchasing one.

Even hot summer nights cool down, and the temperature change alone can trigger an attack for many children. Anticipate the attack and dress your child warmly (don't overdo it though). Keep your child dry, and elevate the head of his bedding slightly. Observe flow meter readings and medicate according to your doctor's instructions.

Prepare foods for the food allergic child at home. Turkey burgers look and cook like hamburgers. Turkey and chicken franks can be substituted for hot dogs. Individual-size packages of cereal can be cut open to make a bowl and fruit juices in individual-size cartons can be substituted for milk.

Simplify special food preparation procedures whenever possible. Wrap allergy-free meals in heavy-duty foil and grill with the family dinner. A seasoned lamb chop, potato and sliced carrots dotted lightly with milk-free margarine or bacon fat, wrapped in heavy-duty foil and grilled will make a tasty dinner (provided your child has the same food allergies as Brooke!).

In choosing a campground, look for one with a nice shower facility with hot and cold running water. Cold morning or evening showers may be disastrous. If your child cannot bathe at the bathhouse after playing all day in the grass, pollen, dust and dirt of Mother Earth, comb or brush your child's hair to remove surface allergens while heating water on the cookstove. When the water becomes warm, not hot, use a washrag (or two) to give your child a sponge bath.

Pack extra inhalers and medicines just in case some of it gets lost. It is difficult to get prescriptions filled in the remote areas that campgrounds are located in, so plan ahead! Pack medications in an airtight, waterproof container. Keep the nebulizer, flow meter and stethoscope in a dry, protected area as well.

SCOUTING

One Girl Scout troop leader told me she was unaware that two of her teenage girls had asthma until one of them was having trouble breathing at the campfire sing-along and another girl tossed her inhaler to her to use. Sharing inhalers is not a good idea, but the point is that the girls' parents had not adequately prepared the Scout leader to handle an asthma attack. Nor had the girls been instructed about sharing medications. You can't expect a Scout leader to know how to help your child if you don't give instructions. Provide written instructions for an emergency situation.

Most Scout leaders are more than willing to help our children reach goals. They don't insist that the child forgo medications or dietary restrictions to earn a badge. Scout leaders, by nature, give generously of themselves and want to see our children be successful. On the other hand, we can't expect the

Scout leader to remind our children to use their inhalers during meetings or to make other Scouts abide by our child's dietary restrictions. Children old enough to participate in Scouts are old enough to remember when they are to use inhalers and which foods to avoid. If necessary, provide allergy-free snacks for your child.

There will most likely be occasions when your child will not be able to participate in a planned Scouting activity. This may include those times when he is recovering from a serious bout with asthma, bronchitis or pneumonia or when the planned activity involves exposure to an allergen that does not respond to pretreatment. Remind your child that there will be other opportunities for fun in the future.

Scouting can be such a positive experience. If you are concerned about your child's health, volunteer to be a Scout leader or to help on special outings or with parties. This is sometimes difficult to do if both parents work, but if Scouting is important to your child and you can find the time, the rewards can be great.

CHAPTER **11**

PLANNING
A FAMILY
VACATION

A VACATION SHOULD BE A TIME OF RELAXATION and freedom from routine, an opportunity to reevaluate priorities and to refuel the mind's creativity. Unfortunately, asthma is no respecter of vacations and holidays. For families that have children with asthma, vacation planning can stir up not only excitement and anticipation, but also anxiety.

Parents of children with asthma must plan vacations very carefully. There are new allergens, activities and changes in climate or altitude to consider. There are medications to buy and equipment to pack. Mode of travel and lodging enroute and at the final destination must also be studied. Vacation planning for the food allergic child also includes menu planning, food storage and preservation.

Though vacation planning can clearly present a challenge, it is a challenge worth accepting and can be accomplished with an organized plan. "Your mission, should you choose to accept it" is to go on vacation and enjoy it without asthma incident and to have a plan of action should asthma flare while away from home. Certainly, we all hope that asthma will not interfere with a long-awaited vacation; however, a plan that includes a strategy for handling asthma attacks increases the likelihood that the vacation will still be a success.

VACATION-PLANNING CHECKLIST

- *Know your destination:* Are you planning a stay at a rustic mountain retreat or a sun-filled beach trip? Will you be visiting friends or relatives who smoke or have pets? Are you traveling during the rainy season? Is the weather expected to be extremely cold or hot? What are the seasonal allergens? Will you be close to a medical facility or will you be isolated from help? Is there only one destination or will there be several stops along the way? Will the vacation time be spent at home as a family or will extended members of the family be visiting? Is your child's vacation time divided between two parents living separately?

- *Activities planned:* Will your vacation include the adventures and excitement of an amusement park, water slides, hiking, skiing? Will it be spent relaxing, fishing or at a family reunion? Is the vacation centered around holiday activities such as Christmas or Thanksgiving?

Vacations usually mean a break from routine and any disturbance in an effective asthma management routine could affect your child's health. Late nights combined with action-packed days are going to weaken the body's already compromised system. People enjoy vacations more if they get enough rest. To protect your vacation, do not deviate from the medication schedule and plan for sufficient rest for a child with asthma.

• *Mode of travel:* Whether you will be traveling by car, plane, train, boat, bus or horse influences what you must do to prepare for a vacation with your child. Children who require several breathing treatments a day should not forgo them while enroute to the destination.

For example, you can rent or buy a nebulizer (if you don't already own one) that can be operated by its own battery or can be plugged into a car cigarette lighter. If your nebulizer does not have this capability, most rest stops have electrical hookups. Remember that at rest stops kids enjoy running around picking up acorns and feathers, chasing each other and getting a snack out of the cooler. The child with asthma needs to have that same opportunity to stretch and play too. That's why I like the portable nebulizers for traveling. Give your child a breathing treatment *before* you pull into the rest stop. Then let all the kids have fun running off energy.

Prepare for air travel by packing a carry-on case with all medications, stethoscope, peak flow meter and the nebulizer (if one has been prescribed). Flights less than two hours are now smoke-free! However, when purchasing tickets for longer flights, try to arrange for seating in the middle portion of the nonsmoking section. This protects your child from "first class" smoke that travels to the front of the no-smoking section and smoke from the coach smokers' section wafting to the front. Avoid "first class" travel because this section of the plane is rarely big enough or its air filtered well enough to accommodate smoking and nonsmoking sections. You may be able to book on an airline that prohibits smoking. (Northwest Orient does this now.)

Portable battery-operated nebulizers are approved for use in airplanes, though the electric units which require a plug cannot be used in flight. I checked this policy with several major airlines before our family flew to Walt Disney World last summer. As it turned out, Brooke did not need a treatment while she was on the plane, but I don't take chances.

The dry air in airplanes can cause a problem for some asthmatics as can pressure changes (particularly for those children with sinus allergies and congestion). Be sure your child has plenty to drink. Chewing gum and frequent yawning help relieve pressure in ears. Ask the doctor ahead of time whether any special premedication (decongestants) will be needed.

- *Lodging:* Will the child need a crib? If so, what kind of mattress does the hotel use? Is it vinyl-covered? Is it more practical for you to provide your baby's bedding? Will you be staying with friends or relatives? If you are staying at a beach cottage or mountain cabin, are you to be the first people to open it for the season? Has a cleaning crew prepared it for your arrival? Rodent droppings and urine, musty molds and dust are common in vacation dwellings.

Whether you are obtaining the rental through an agency or through a friend, be certain the cabin will be cleaned before you get there.

Most large hotels have very clean rooms and some have entire floors designated for nonsmokers. Many bargain-basement hotels are sufficient, but some have dusty, musty-smelling rooms and mattresses. Try to examine the room before paying the clerk. Also check the room's air-conditioner filter (if accessible) and check room air vents for cobwebs. You might even want to take a small portable air cleaner along.

• *Food:* Parents of children who have asthma and food allergies often become discouraged when planning vacation menus because what is easy to prepare at home is usually more complicated on the road. The meal planner must consider where each of three meals a day plus snacks will be eaten. Foods which must be protected from spoilage will require special packaging.

Individual-size containers of "safe foods" pack neatly into backpacks or purses, just in case the restaurant menu does not include the foods your child can eat. Most waiters are very nice and do not complain if your child must eat his cereal with apple juice instead of milk. There are exceptions, though, and much to our disappointment we encountered one who was rather put out by Brooke's breakfast cereal and juice. Rather than create a public scene, we waited until he went away and explained to Brooke that his ignorance was showing. We all agreed that it was a shame that he had such bad manners.

Parents also need to consider the feelings of their food-allergic little ones. The milk-allergic child can't be expected to get excited about a family trip to the ice cream store if he is going to come away empty-handed. A quick trip to a 7-Eleven for a Slurpee or a popsicle (with all the "ceremony" of the ice cream store) can solve the problem of hurt feelings.

If you will be traveling by air, most airlines will prepare special food trays if you call ahead of time.

• *Finances:* Vacations can be fun whether they cost thousands of dollars or next to nothing. One thing is certain, taking an uncontrolled asthmatic on vacation will be costly. Not only will it involve the expenses of extra medications or emergency room visits but asthma can cut the entire trip short. Bring appropriate health insurance forms and identification so that you don't have to use vacation money to pay for medical services.

• *Length of vacation:* How long do you plan to be away from home? Extended vacations require far more advanced planning than short ones. When parents travel with young children with asthma (especially when asthma is not yet controlled), I usually recommend short trips over long weekends. Routines are disturbed only mildly and are easy to reestablish upon return. Each time you venture away, you pick up information and confidence to make the next trip longer and more fun.

Plan ahead and take time to find viable answers to each potential trouble area. Advance planning always helps make things run smoothly. However, if you get a spur of the moment phone call, as we did from friends vacationing on the beach in Duck, North Carolina, inviting you for an almost free four days of fun and sun, pack fast and have a great time. But don't do what we did. Dale and I packed suitcases, foods, meds, filled the gas tank, checked the oil and lights and fastened our seat belts. Dale said, "I've got the nebulizer." I said, "I've got the medicines," and at 4 A.M. we pulled out of the driveway without the masking and tubing to run the nebulizer!

PACKING LIST

- Pack all medications in a shoe box, cosmetic case or similar container and keep it accessible at all times. Put a brightly colored strip of tape across the top to make it easy to identify.

- As you are packing the medications, think about various situations that trigger attacks and the medications you will need to stop them. An attack triggered by a bee sting requires a different procedure from an attack triggered by exercise. It is far better to pack more medication than you expect to use than to be away from home trying to get a prescription filled. But there's no need to draw attention to or make an issue of packing all the medications. Pack them as you would the suntan lotion or bug repellent. Label the container and load it in the car.

- Store a *summarized* copy of your child's medical history inside the box containing the medications and keep another in your purse or wallet, so in the event of an accident, medical personnel will be aware of medical problems. Also, the MedAlert (available through most local pharmacies) makes identification medallions and bracelets that convey vital medical information.

- Don't forget the insurance membership cards.

- One person should be in charge of packing all medications and equipment. Don't forget the flow meter, the stethoscope or the nebulizer with the masking and tubing.

- Regularly scheduled daily medications can be organized and packed into small sandwich Ziploc bags or special containers. However, an extra set of meds should be packed separately, just in case something happens to the primary container.

- When touring involves a lot of walking, school-age children can carry their own inhaler in a backpack with their drinks and snacks. A parent should also carry a spare, just in case the youngster loses the backpack.

- When traveling by air always pack all meds (stethoscope, flow meter and nebulizer included) in a carry-on bag and keep it with you. Under no circumstances should you check this baggage in at the ticket counter. The Dura Neb 2000 portable nebulizer has plenty of room in its carry bag for a stethoscope, flow meter, nebulizer meds and attachments. The carry bag looks like a camera bag: it is lightweight, durable and inconspicuous. DeVilbiss also makes a very lightweight portable worth checking out. See the Resources section.

OTHER TIPS

- Two months before you plan to leave for vacation, visit with your child's primary asthma management doctor for a health assessment and a prevention plan to carry you through vacation. This gives you plenty of time to clear up any conditions which may be beginning to flare. It also allows you to get a head start on strengthening the health of your child before vacation has the chance to weaken it.

- If visiting a large family amusement park such as Walt Disney World, bring or rent a stroller for children under four years old. They tire quickly when they have to match four of their steps to our one. When they tire, they get cranky, which can actually play a role in triggering an episode. Strollers offer a place to pack snacks and extra drinks and meds, too.

- Another amusement park idea is to wear a backpack (or have your child wear it) with extra drinks and snacks packed inside. That way the food allergic child always has something to snack on. Children without food allergies are likely to ask for equal treatment! Include a sweater even on hot days. The temperature change involved in walking from the hot sun into an air-conditioned restaurant or theater is enough to trigger asthma in some children. Please don't take children with (or without) asthma under four years of age to places such as Walt Disney World unless it is off season and cool and you don't mind giving your child a chance to rest often. We saw more families fighting and babies crying because the *parents* wanted to go to Walt Disney World. It was sad to see children so tired that they couldn't enjoy an ice cream cone while watching the beautiful Electric Parade or the Fourth of July fireworks display.

- If a winter holiday involves sledding or skiing, watch over the child with asthma. Plodding through the snow is hard work, and the cold air can trigger bronchoconstriction. Children should keep their faces covered, have an inhaler handy and always be accompanied by a responsible partner. (A 3M air warming mask can be worn under a ski mask or scarf without embarrassment. See Resources section, Products, under Biotech Systems.)

- Schedule rest periods each day. To avoid argument, establish the schedule at the beginning of the day. "This morning after breakfast, we will all hop in the van and drive to the lake and swim until just after lunch. Then we'll come back home and take a rest, eat an early dinner and go to the county fair afterward. How's that sound?" You may hear an objection or two but a commitment to consistency at the beginning of the vacation will be rewarded throughout.

- If an activity will bring exposure to an allergen—such as a trip to the county fair, the circus or an amusement park— ask your doctor about pretreatments. Pretreatments are safe when doctor's orders are followed. I like to think of pretreatments as the rubber glove treatment. Rubber gloves protect your hands and manicure from hot water and abrasive chemicals. Pretreatments protect your child's lungs and the vacation fun.

- Locate the emergency room nearest to your final destination (and at various points along the way if traveling by car) before you leave home. The hotel concierge or your travel agent can help you obtain this information. If your child requires a *specific* procedure for emergency treatment (such as oxygen with breathing treatments and adrenaline injections), ask your doctor to write instructions (using his letterhead stationery) for the attending emergency-room physician.

- Inform your doctor at least six months in advance if you are planning to take your child abroad. This gives your doctor an opportunity to help you plan prevention and emergency tactics. In other countries, medical treatment for asthma is often very different from that in the United States. Also allow plenty of time for scheduling immunizations if needed.

- There may or may not be any need to carry a nebulizer compressor with your child everywhere you go. Usually, keeping it accessible (as in a locked car, in an insulated zipper bag if it is very hot or very cold) will keep it close enough.

- If your children start to get overheated, tired or hungry, duck into an air-conditioned display or museum long enough to cool off, get a drink of water, discuss plans to eat and then head back to the hotel for a rest. Don't expend their energies. It is their vacation, too.

Vacation planning can cause anxious feelings if you are not prepared. Sometimes, even when you are prepared, the plans go astray. I remember one vacation several years ago, when we spent the July 4th holiday at a rustic cabin in Gettysburg. The cabin had not been used for a while and, though it was neat, a layer of dust, mold and mildew had settled. The kids played on a rope swing hanging from an old tree in the backyard while Dale and I opened up the doors and windows (which only added pollen to the list of allergens) and mopped and dusted. Just about the time we finished unpacking, we heard Brooke crying. In an attempt to make the swing go higher, her brother's last push smacked her into the side of the tree. A couple of scrapes and bruises would have been the only injuries if the tree hadn't been covered with poison ivy, to which Brooke is extremely allergic. We bathed her right away but the damage was already done.

Two days later, in the smoldering July heat and humidity, we visited a battlefield encampment, a special reenactment to celebrate Independence Day. The men were marching in a drill when suddenly, about a dozen horsemen rode onto the field. A gentle breeze wafted just enough "horse air" as Brooke called it, to make her already trigger-happy asthma get started. She and I went back to the van to sit in the shade for a breathing treatment and a dose of antihistamines while Dale and the boys took the trail to the campsite displays. Ten minutes later, we set off in search of them. Thinking Brooke was at my side, I was enjoying the displays as I looked for my family. Brooke, thinking I was at her side, was enjoying a totally different set of displays. Imagine my surprise when I found Brooke before I found Dale or the boys. She'd befriended an "injured soldier" at the Red Cross tent in front of which was a smoky campfire.

The sum total of all the allergens meant Brooke's asthma flared for the entire vacation. Thankfully, we were able to continue our activities without emergency room visits or hospitalizations, but only because we had a doctor-prescribed plan and we were able to keep a good humor (most of the time) about things. As soon as we returned home, Brooke's asthma improved and our lives quickly returned to normal.

Depending on the severity and frequency of your child's health problems, vacation planning can be a lot of work. Some of you will need to do more preparation than others. However, it helps to put all this extra effort into proper perspective. Make a decision to have fun on the trip despite the hassles you have to overcome and it will be worth the effort. Allow plenty of time to make all the necessary preparations and things should run pretty smoothly. The rewards are great and our children are young for such a short time. So are we, really. Make each day count and make fond memories.

CHAPTER 12

ASTHMA IS
A FAMILY
AFFAIR

H E COULD HEAR THEM ARGUE EVEN THOUGH HE WAS *in his room and they were in theirs. They thought he was sleeping and he wished he could. Instead, he lay in his bed clutching his "forbidden" rag of a teddy bear catching tears with the corner of his pillowcase as he listened to his parents fighting again.*

"You don't understand! You have got to let the boy alone!"

"Me? I'm not the one who tells him he can't play ball or

won't let him outside to play with his friends! No! I'm not the one who has turned our son into a wimp . . ."

"Sh-h-h! *He might hear you! And he is* not *a wimp! He just can't do the things you want him to do because he can't breathe!* He has asthma! *If he were blind, would you call him a wimp if he didn't want to try out for the basketball team?"*

"Well, take him to another doctor then. Get someone who can fix his asthma. You just accept him the way he is so he won't ever want to be anything else other than sick. I am sick of his being sick!"

"You think I like this? I had to quit my job to stay home and take care of him. I'm sorry. I don't mean it the way it sounds, but it's like you are blaming me for his asthma. I can't believe you don't understand how he feels. You had asthma when you were a kid. Don't you remember?"

"Yeah. I do remember that I played with my friends like everyone else and I grew out of it. So, do you want to blame his asthma on me? I didn't die. I did fine. I'm not a wimp."

The door slammed. His mother was crying, and so was he. He wanted to get out of bed and hug her but he felt sick to his stomach. He loved his father and his mother, but it seemed all they did now was fight about his asthma. "If I were a girl," he thought, "they wouldn't be fighting." And sometimes he did wish he had another doctor. Not that he liked going to see the doctor, but he knew he wasn't getting any better and he was getting tired, too tired to keep working so hard to breathe.

Sleep finally came. Morning's light beckoned him to a breakfast of cereal and "wimp" pills and syrup medicines. His mother poured his father's coffee in silence while he was ignored by his father, hidden behind the morning newspaper. How he hated those pills. How he hated having asthma!

"Tryouts for basketball are next week. I think I'd like to give it a try. Okay?"

The corner of the newspaper dipped in his mother's direction. Her face was swollen from crying the night before but as her worn expression changed to anxiety, he knew in an instant he'd asked the wrong question.

"Well, it's up to your father," she said, and turned away.

His father folded the newspaper and placed it alongside his plate and he said, "I don't know, son. Do you think you can do it with your asthma?"

Anger burned inside him and without thinking he blurted, "Why don't you just say it? Why don't you just say what you think . . . That I can't do it because I am such a WIMP! WIMP! WIMP! WIMP!" He pushed away from the table because he could feel his chest tightening up again. He hated his chest. As he backed out of the kitchen and before turning down the hall, he angrily shouted, "AND I HATE YOU!"

In a family, one person does not hurt without the other members hurting too. Sometimes this hurt is shown as compassion, or denial, or even anger. Asthma does not have to be life-threatening to affect the family, only chronic. The adversity caused by asthma does not have to cripple the family. When responded to properly, adversity can actually draw families close together.

In this chapter, we will look at asthma's impact on the home in several areas. Remember that the period between diagnosis and control is often the most difficult time, and for most of our children, that is only a temporary period. The key to keeping a positive, productive attitude during this time is to work toward the day when the bad days will be only a bad memory.

SIBLING RIVALRY

The *MA Report* mail bag received an anonymous letter from a woman whose sister has asthma. The letter expressed resentment, hurt and even anger that during their childhood, her sister had received so much attention while she and her brother had been "ignored." A few days later, she called to talk and get things off her mind. After our phone conversation, it was easy to see why she still felt a sense of betrayal and abandonment, even though she is now an adult with children of her own. Tangled feelings were released as we discussed her past, and we both grew in understanding of asthma's impact on the family.

She said more attention had been devoted to her sister. She described having to do more than her share of the household chores because her sister was too sick to help. She said her brother and she would be spanked if they misbehaved but her sister's actions were never corrected for fear that she would have an attack.

As I listened to her, I tried to put myself in her parents' position twenty years ago when asthma-out-of-control was the norm. What a frightening and frustrating way for a family to live. Asthma-out-of-control is such a consuming disease. It eats up family-together time. It demands immediate attention regardless of any other circumstance or event. And the more restrictions asthma places on the family, the more tempting it is to shift the blame for everyone's problems on the child who has asthma.

Parents often try to compensate for the frailty of their child with material gifts and fewer responsibilities. Frequent doctor visits, hospitalizations and emergency room treatments are sometimes viewed by siblings as special treatment. They feel the asthmatic sibling has power over the other members of the family.

The adult who shared her story with me offered this insight: "If only my parents had explained what was going on! Instead, whenever my sister had an attack, my brother and I were sent to the other room to watch TV and stay. I would have liked to help but when I offered, I was told I could help by doing dishes. I would have liked to have been part of the solution. Instead, I felt like I was in the way."

Adversity in the home can surprisingly become the cement that bonds a family together. It doesn't have to tear people and families apart. We must make family unity an objective. Then we will begin to see the ways we can creatively involve family members in part of the solution, teach discipline and divide chores evenly and according to ability. Though it is difficult in any family, try to remember to distribute attention to all children equally. Otherwise, our children may grow up to find they have nothing in common but rivalry.

MARRIAGE AND DIVORCE

Physically and emotionally, the child needs to have his parents focus on finding a solution to his health concerns. But when divorce strikes the family, his needs become secondary. The parents are understandably preoccupied with the heartbreak and suffering involved with the separation.

Certainly no one involved needs the added stress of a chronic illness at a time like this.

Often, divorce affects parents' perception of a child's asthma because their ability to deal with additional stress is overloaded. Suddenly, every attack is suspected of being faked (sometimes it truly is, but it should not be ignored regardless). The child may view himself as a great burden, and maybe even as the reason for his family's unhappiness. Siblings may blame the separation on the child with asthma. Family counselors and pediatricians may suddenly associate the asthma, which has raged out of control for years, with the stress of the broken family. The deeper they dig into the psychological, the less likely it becomes that they discover the real source of trouble.

Stress does not cause asthma, but it can trigger an attack in someone who has asthma. Stress triggers chemical changes in the body. When the body's chemical balance gets tipped, some people who have asthma will start wheezing. They can't do any more about a stress trigger than they can about allergens.

You see your child every day. If his asthma has not been triggered by emotions in the past, or if it has not worsened through parental separation, don't go blaming your failed marriage for your child's asthma. Deal with his feelings about the divorce or separation and deal with his asthma. Don't add to his frustrations by not understanding that the two can coexist without causing each other.

If you take a moment to reflect, you will have a good idea whether your child's asthma is being worsened by family stress. Does your child's asthma tend to improve, worsen or remain the same when visiting the parent who left home? If your child gets better, is it because your former spouse has a more allergy-free environment? Could it be that the ex is medicating the child more in line with the doctor's instructions? If not, is the child under less stress when with the other spouse?

If your child's asthma gets worse when visiting your ex-partner could it be that medications are ignored and preventive methods of management are relaxed? Does the ex believe the asthma would improve if the child were better disciplined? Does the child leave an allergy-free environment for a less protected one? Or is your child so desperate to bring his parents back together that she purposely exposes herself to allergens to induce an attack which she hopes will bring you together, even if it is only at the hospital bedside?

Divorce and asthma are two high-stress problems which are competing for your attention. Regardless of how you feel, you have a child who needs you. Take time to work through the pain of divorce and separation constructively, and not at your child's expense.

If you and your spouse are considering separation or divorce and you have a child with asthma, if there is any way to restore a working, loving relationship, do it. Otherwise, you both have your work cut out for you. Here are just a few of the questions which will need answers:

- Who is going to take financial responsibility for medical bills?

- Who is going to take primary responsibility for taking the child to the doctor, learning about triggers and early warning signals?

- Who will be responsible for teaching the child appropriate self-management skills?

- Are both parents willing to support the child with the same asthma information? If so, the parents need to be able to *communicate well with each other.*

- Are both parents willing to take allergy-proofing steps in the child's environment in both of her homes?

- Are both parents willing to medicate responsibly when the child is in his or her care?

- Do both parents have a working knowledge of methods of prevention and what to do in case of an emergency?

- Do stepparents complain about having to make "severe adjustments" or shy away from responsibility for the child's health?

- Are diet restrictions respected at both homes?

- Is the child expected to behave responsibly at both homes, especially concerning age-appropriate self-management of asthma?

- Does one parent insist that the child's asthma is all in the head without providing for and participating in family counseling? (In other words, if this is the accusation, what steps does he or she suggest to remedy the situation? Is he or she willing to participate in the solution?)

- Does one parent, stepparent or even grandparent try to insist on folklore remedies such as the myth that the child should be left alone because he will grow out of it?

- How does your child perceive her role in this divorce?

There is no doubt that some family situations are improved in the absence of a destructive spouse. Some ex-partners have problems with substance abuse or emotional disturbances. Many ex-partners refuse to set aside their bitterness or self-interest to consider the physical needs of their children.

Some people claim that asthma was responsible for breaking up their marriage. More than likely, the marriage would have toppled due to any adversity. Asthma just happened to be handy.

Indeed, asthma can bring out the worst in our personalities if it is raging out of control. When we don't get enough sleep, or when one spouse shoulders the entire burden for the child's health care without any support or encouragement from the other, pressures start to build and weakened foundations begin to crumble.

Few families have the luxury of disbanding under friendly circumstances. But regardless of the negative feelings one parent has for the other, the temptation to use their child and his asthma as a weapon or pawn should be resisted.

If your marriage is under strain from asthma, get the asthma under control and spend some time with a quality marriage counselor. Learn how to communicate effectively. Remember, the stresses of asthma are few when the asthma is under control.

SINGLE-PARENTING THE ASTHMATIC CHILD

The game plan for single-parenting the child with asthma is the same as for everyone else; it's just that the entire burden for the health and well-being of the child falls on the shoulders of one person.

I was widowed four days before my second son was born. I was lonely and scared. I doubted my ability to raise my children, but even more, I doubted the ability of any man to love me and my two boys the way we needed to be loved. God proved His great compassion for me and gave me a wonderful man, a mate far more perfect than I would ever have dreamed to ask for. Dale and I have been married just over eleven years now and I am thankful to God for every day we share together. But those three years alone were excruciating. I know what it feels like to be a single parent and I know what it is like to have a child with asthma but for me, thankfully, the two did not coincide with each other. Though things may seem tough, God's compassion is greater than your need and will sustain you as you rally your support.

Single parents of children who have asthma should expand their support system. It helps to have a network of friends because asthma's demands on the family drain a person quickly, particularly one who is alone.

Enlist the help of your parents, other family members, church friends, neighbors, even a teacher at school. For example, one young mother called me because she was in need of a special crib for her son. She was very poor and was renting a single room in a house shared by another family. There was only enough space for a bed and a dresser and a collapsible crib. The crib had to collapse or the mother would not have been able to walk through the room without stepping on her bed.

There were other problems too. The girl was unmarried and the father of the child did not help with medical expenses. The girl had little education and found it hard to find a job that offered medical insurance. To complicate matters even more, she could not find a baby-sitter who was willing to watch her child because the baby demanded a lot of medical attention.

She was exasperated and felt she had no place to turn. I talked to her about mobilizing resources. I asked her if she belonged to a church. She said she had just started attending one in the area. I suggested she make an appointment to speak with the minister and discuss her problem. Many churches offer temporary support to members who are in need due to unusual circumstances. For example, churches often have "clothing closets" for the needy which would alleviate her need to purchase clothing for her baby and herself.

She had already contacted the state and local social services departments. Evidently, her family had somewhat disowned her since she'd had the baby so they could not be relied upon at this time for help, but we talked about the people in her neighborhood with whom she might want to exchange services. Would she be willing to iron clothes for someone who could watch her baby three mornings a week . . . and so on.

Another mother I talked to has twins with asthma. Her ex-husband offers no support and, though he has asthma, denies its existence in his children.

The asthmatic stepmother of a child with asthma was distraught that the child's natural parents (the child's natural mother was the single parent) both deny that the child has asthma. The list of potential problems in single parenting increases greatly when parents or blended families cannot agree on the health needs of the child with asthma.

Single parents should make a list of seemingly insurmountable problems and then find a way to tackle them creatively one at a time. You will have to be more creative to accomplish some of the things on your list than if you had the committed assistance of a loving spouse, but controlled asthma is still a possibility.

PART-TIME SINGLE PARENTING

Some of you have spouses whose jobs require travel. It is difficult for husbands or wives to provide the emotional support needed when they are many miles away and when they are gone for extended periods of time. Many times, the absent parent finds it difficult to comprehend the intensity of the burden.

Traveling spouses are obviously in no position to be of any immediate help when they are miles from home, but it doesn't mean they don't care and aren't anxious while away. Demonstrating that care when returning home is probably going to be too late because the crisis will be over.

The traveling parent can offer a sense of stability and presence in the home by remaining accessible and understanding. A phone call to your child at the hospital or at home will reassure him that you care. A phone discussion with the child's doctor will show the doctor, your spouse and your child that you care. A follow-up phone call to the asthma-managing spouse will also be appreciated.

The stay-at-home parent can create a welcoming atmosphere for the traveling parent upon return even in the middle of asthma upheaval. Though your life may be controlled by many do's and don't's, timed medications and treatments, etc., the traveling spouse needs time to adjust. If you have not been communicating well with the spouse while he was absent, do not expect him to understand what is going on in your life as soon as he walks through the door.

Traveling parents need to be open and perceptive because the stay-at-home parent may be under tremendous pressure. Whenever possible, it is a good idea for the stay-at-home parent to take a "break," i.e., go visit relatives or a friend for the weekend. It provides a refreshing change and allows the parent who is frequently absent to experience the responsibilities and rewards of twenty-four-hour child care.

One mother I talked to recently said that her husband was very complacent about their son's asthma. She said he felt asthma was not "macho" and his way of coping with it was to ignore it. The mother, an asthmatic, recognized that the only way to raise a "macho" asthmatic was to get asthma under control. The father came home only on weekends and saw very little of the impact asthma had made in the lives of his family. Since he did not understand, he could not offer the love and support his wife and son needed. He shut out that major part of their lives.

This mother said she was having some progress in dealing with the problem by suggesting that asthma wasn't all bad. She said she almost felt sorry for her husband, that he was missing such a wonderful opportunity to show support in a loved one's time of need. She said, "There is a relationship that forms and bonds during those wee hours of the morning, during the wait in the doctor's office or emergency room, as your child cries out his or her own frustrations at being "different." You can read that child like a book. You may bear the burdens but you also witness the triumphs." Then she added, "We need to look not at what we have lost, but at what we have gained." This is a mother who really wants to make her marriage work.

WHEN BOTH PARENTS WORK

In today's society, families with two working parents are as common as families with two working cars. Regardless of whether a two-income family is a matter of choice or need, if your child has asthma, adjustments will have to be made.

If asthma is a rare occurrence, it is probably a part of life you take in stride. If your child has more than three asthma flares a year, life is probably a bit more complicated. If your child's asthma is severe or out of control, the impact on the two-income family will be especially great. Part of the reason for this is that asthma is an exhausting, time-consuming disease, and working parents already have enough stress in their lives without asthma.

You will have to work to bring life back into balance. If your idea of balance means both parents work, then your goal will be to gain control over the asthma as quickly as possible so that you will be able to accomplish this goal. This may mean that you take a leave of absence or quit your job temporarily to concentrate on asthma management rather than fearing "the phone call" at work each day.

Many parents cannot afford to give up the second income. After all, asthma expenses put a crunch on the family budget. Other parents feel that their career would suffer a setback and that they have worked too hard to let it fall apart at this time. They may have to enlist the help of family members or the services of a full–time nanny.

Even though the decision to work or take a leave of absence can be most difficult, it is one that only you can make.

It may help to make a list of all the asthma-related concerns you have. On a separate sheet of paper, make a list of the reasons why you work. On a third sheet of paper, list the personal stresses you are under.

The first two lists are self-explanatory. The third list is the humdinger. Put the kids to bed before making this list; you'll need some solitude to look at your life objectively. This list should answer the following questions:

- What are my responsibilities to my family? To myself? To my job? (These include financial obligations, personal goals, etc.)
- Am I as healthy as I used to be?
- Am I too tired to enjoy my family?
- Have I lost time to listen to my children? My spouse?
- Am I so tired at night that I literally fall into bed exhausted?
- Do I like what I see when I look in the mirror? (You *know* what I mean!)
- Have I lost/gained too much weight?
- Is it a struggle to get my grocery shopping and other errands completed?
- Am I satisfied that I give my job and my home my best?

Each two-income family that includes a child with a chronic illness must take personal inventory from time to time. Guided by these three lists, you can make a wise decision. Quitting work is not to be equated with failure. Nor is it to be considered the only option or the "right" thing to do.

Staying at work is not a sentence to feeling guilty. You are not always faced with an "either/or" situation and decisions such as these don't have to be final. Before making major career changes, examine your asthma management plan. Changing your lifestyle because your child is sick is a noble gesture, but may not be the solution to a situation which ultimately needs concentrated doses of medical attention.

One mom wrote that she'd had forty-one jobs in nine years. She said her employers would be understanding until she missed so much time that her work started piling up. Then they would have to face the reality that the job required someone who could be more dependable. There are other families of children who have asthma in which both mother and father have successful, fulfilling careers. But just because they are able to be successful at both doesn't mean they have it easy.

Two-income families must have the devotion and commitment of the entire family to make it work. Efforts to allergy-proof the child's bedroom, vacuum and dust more frequently, drive him to the doctor for allergy shots and still involve him in activities such as sports or Scouts require squeezing many things into the few hours you have left at the end of the day. This kind of time crunching takes family co-operation.

Creative alternatives to the standard two-income family are also available. Don't overlook income-producing talents that can be exercised at home. Sometimes it takes an adversity that pins us in our homes to discover hidden talents and resources. Gail Jenkins of Tehachapi, California, whose daughter Mimi has an asthma history very similar to Brooke's, is an artist who started a home business actually inspired by Mimi's asthma:

> *I am an artist, so when Mimi first started having problems at age one, I would design and make her little stuffed toys. My husband suggested I market the pat-*

terns by mail order since I was homebound with Mimi, for what seemed like would be forever. So I did, and it has done well for me. I have kept the business small so I don't need to hire help. Mimi helps "when she's in the mood" by counting eyes, noses, etc. I hope she'll take more interest as she gets older. It helps pay for those little extras—especially Mimi's medication, which runs close to $75 a month now.

When we have family goals and objectives, we tend to strengthen each other. Then when the crisis period is over, we will be all the closer because of it.

AFTERWORD:
LOOKING FORWARD

When uncontrolled asthma consumes our lives, we soon forget the freedom of laughter, the joy of taking a walk on a summer afternoon and the thrill of watching our children grow up. When asthma grips the family, it is difficult to balance our protector role and give our children the freedom they need to explore and expand their world.

Asthma's impact on the child is greatest, I believe, when the child becomes aware that he is different. Most six-year-olds do not require pills, nebulizer treatments or a special lunch at school every day. Most twelve-year-olds do not have to take pills and puff medication before attending the seventh-grade dance. Most seventeen-year-olds can outdistance their grandmothers in a leg race. Not so for many children growing up with uncontrolled asthma. These children look around and know that they are different.

Asthma's side effects grow proportionately more cumbersome with each day it is left raging out of control. Children whose asthma is under control know and accept that their bodies require special treatment. These children understand that they are different, but not part of a freak show. They realize that the best asthma attack is one that is prevented.

They have choices to make and they grow up accustomed to making responsible decisions.

That doesn't mean they enjoy the breathing treatments, nose sprays or inhalers. It doesn't mean that they won't complain about things from time to time. It does mean that ultimately they are able to accept the fact that their management program enables them to be the most that they want to be.

For those of you who are still struggling, I want so badly to reach out of the final pages of this book, take your hand and tell you in person that a better day is coming. Right now, you are the grown-up voice of a child in pain. You would like nothing more than to erase the suffering or even take it all on yourself.

Even so, these days will pass and as you work toward the goal of asthma under control, life with asthma will become less stressful. And though the period between diagnosis and control may linger longer than you'd like, there will be plenty of occasion for smiles.

Though asthma may have you feeling that you are in a bottomless pit with no means of escape, take heart! I won't tell you that it will be easy, but if you persevere you, too, can reduce the impact of asthma in your life. Asthma attacks may be controlling your life right now, but that will change. It's time to attack the asthma!

Learning to control asthma is a little like doing a giant jig-

MOTHERS AND CHILDREN

Being the mom of three "wheezers" has its light moments too! My boys love music and love to drum along with tapes. One afternoon, my two-year-old turned a trash can upside down, sat on a Tupperware container and began drumming with two rulers. I said, "Benj, why don't you get your teddy bear? He'd love to listen to you." He looked at me

saw puzzle. In the beginning you have a pile of seemingly unrelated pieces. Where do you begin? You start with the obvious. Sort through the pieces until you find the ones that look like they might form the border. Take a closer look and try to match two of those pieces to give you something to build on. The going is slow at first. It takes a lot of sifting and sorting just to find two components that fit. As you progress it gets easier. Occasionally you hit a snag. No matter how hard you look at that pile of pieces, you just can't find one that fits. But then someone with a fresh viewpoint comes along, takes one look and the very piece you've been searching for seems to catch his eye. Once that piece is found, others seem to fall easily into place.

Here are a few suggestions to help you get started piecing the asthma control puzzle together:

with a very puzzled look, found his teddy bear and held him up to his chest as he began taking deep breaths! I wanted to laugh and cry at the same time, but instead I hugged him and said, "No silly—not your lungs, your drums!" He smiled and went about the serious business of drumming. I will treasure that memory in my heart always.—A mother from Medina, New York

David has asthma triggered by colds. Though the burden of asthma may be heavy at the moment, a better day is coming. After years of trial and error and many different meds, we do have all his many food allergies and asthma under control. We still battle the eczema on a daily basis (it's virtually gone in the summer) with creams and ointments. David has an older sister and often wonders why she does not have any allergies, asthma or eczema. Thanks to the support of our friends and family, hopefully David will endure his school years without many problems and keep enjoying soccer and swimming.—A mother from Topeka, Kansas

- Talk to your doctor. Express your concerns and work to overcome them.

- Keep a daily diary. Record symptoms; suspected triggers and early warning signals; record the medications you use and their effect. A written record helps to organize your thoughts and to pinpoint important information.

- Use a peak flow meter. This is probably the most valuable home diagnostic tool for any asthmatic over the age of four. In the beginning, record peak flow readings at least twice daily. The results will enable both you and your doctor to better visualize the pattern of your child's asthma.

- Take an objective look at your home and lifestyle. Make any necessary changes to rid them of allergens and irritants.

- If you're feeling overwhelmed, find someone to talk to. You are not alone. Countless others are experiencing your same fears and frustrations. Often it helps just to talk to someone who understands your feelings: look for a support group; ask your doctor or nurse to put you in touch with someone who has lived with asthma; call Mothers of Asthmatics or Lung Line.

Asthma can be well controlled! A better day is coming. Go for it!

RESOURCES

Books and Pamphlets

Asthma and Allergy Books

Asthma: The Complete Guide to Self-Management of Asthma and Allergies for Patients and their Families by Allan M. Weinstein, M.D. (hardcover, McGraw-Hill, 1987, $17.95; paperback, Fawcett, 1988, $4.95). If you have only one asthma and allergy book on your shelf, make it this one. It is well organized, easily understood and accurate. No wonder it is a bestseller!

Children with Asthma: A Manual for Parents by Thomas Plaut, M.D., 2nd ed. (Pedipress, Inc., 1988) This popular book gives valuable information for parents of children who have asthma. Recently revised. In bookstores $11.95, or order direct from Pedipress, Inc., 125 Red Gate Lane, Amherst, MA 01002 for $12.95 (book-rate postage included) or $13.95 (UPS or airmail).

The Complete Book of Children's Allergies by B. Robert Feldman, M.D., with David Carroll (Times Books, 1986). A great parent reference guide. Excellent resource section. Also has a wonderful appendix, glossary and section on asthma. $17.95.

Peak Performance: A Strategy for Asthma Self-Assessment by Guillermo Mendoza, M.D. (Mendoza, 1988). This physician's manual is the most detailed guide to optimal peak flow meter use. Order through Mothers of Asthmatics, Inc. 5316 Summit Drive, Fairfax, VA 22030 for $10 plus $1.00 for shipping and handling.

Just for Kids

The Asthma Attack by Charlotte Casterline, M.D. (Info-All Book Company, 1988). A young boy's emergency room experience. Info-All Book Company, 5 Old Wells Lane, Dallas, PA 18612

C.A.L.M.—Childhood Asthma: Learning to Manage—is a program for doctor/parent/child communication. Instruction manuals are geared toward the needs of each as they seek to communicate asthma information. For more information contact the Asthma and Allergy Foundation of America, 1717 Massachusetts Avenue, Washington, D.C. 20036 (202-265-0265).

Captain America Fights the Asthma Monster (Marvel Comics Group, 1987). Asthma education Captain America style! Captain America reveals to children that he, too, had asthma as a child and that asthma can indeed be fought and controlled. Comics are *free* through your physician's Glaxo representative or order direct from Allen & Hanburys division of Glaxo, Inc., 5 Moore Drive, Research Triangle Park, NC 27709. Free.

Captain Wonderlung. An instructional comic book detailing breathing exercises that is available in English, Spanish and French from the American Academy of Pediatrics, 141 Northwest Point Boulevard, Elk Grove Village, IL 60009. Send $1.25 to the attention of Captain Wonderlung at the above address.

Luke Has Asthma, Too by Alison Rogers (Waterfront Books, 1987). A gentle story of two boys who have asthma. Reassures children that asthma can be controlled in a calm manner. Waterfront Books, Burlington, VT 05401. $6.95.

My Friend Has Asthma by Charlotte Casterline, M.D. (Info-All Book Company, 1985). A story for very young children about asthma. Info-All Book Company, 5 Old Wells Lane, Dallas, PA 18612. $4.95.

Sam the Allergen by Charlotte Casterline, M.D. (Info-All Book Company, 1985). What happens when the family pet is also an allergen. Info-All Book Company, 5 Old Wells Lane, Dallas, PA 18612. $4.95.

So You Have Asthma, Too by Nancy Sander (Glaxo, Inc., 1988). This colorful children's book is all about growing up with asthma from the perspective of seven-year-old Brooke Sander. Warmly informative and optimistic. Mothers of Asthmatics, Inc., 10875 Main Street #210, Fairfax, VA 22030. $3.00.

Teaching Myself About Asthma by Guy Parcel, Ph.D., Kathy Tiernan, M.S., Philip Nader, M.D., and Lawrence Weiner, M.D. (Health Education Associates, 1984). An excellent workbook written for children nine to twelve, with notes to family members. 152 pages— paperback. Order by mail from Health Education Associates, 14 North Lake Road, Columbia, SC 29223 (803-765-9233). $9.95 prepaid.

Handbooks

A User's Guide to Peak Flow Monitoring by Guillermo Mendoza, M.D., Nancy Sander and Debbie Scherrer (Mothers of Asthmatics, Inc., 1988). Introduction to peak flow monitoring. This handbook contains all the how-to's of peak flow monitoring and answers your peak flow questions. It can be ordered through Mothers of Asthmatics, Inc., 10875 Main Street #210, Fairfax, VA 22030. $3.00.

The Asthma Organizer by Nancy Sander, Debbie Scherrer and Martha White, M.D. (Mothers of Asthmatics, Inc., 1988). This three-ring-binder system offers a method for tracking your child's daily symptoms, peak flow rates, doctor's office visits and medication information. *The Asthma Organizer* helps coordinate the care of your child at home and at school. It also has a special section for your child's own management plan. This system is used by doctors and their patients at the National Institutes of Health, Bethesda, Maryland, as well as in doctors' offices across the country. It can be ordered through Mothers of Asthmatics, Inc., 10875 Main Street #210, Fairfax, VA 22030. $25 (members of Mothers of Asthmatics, Inc., $17).

Pamphlets and Brochures

Asthma—Episodes and Treatment by Jules Saltman. Public Affairs Pamphlet No. 608, 381 Park Avenue South, New York, NY 10016. Single copies are free.

Asthma: Fact and Fiction; Dust 'n' Stuff; Weeds 'n' Things are three free booklets available through the National Foundation for Asthma, Tucson Medical Center, P.O. Box 30069, Tucson, AZ 85751-0069.

A Patient's Guide to Asthma by Fred Leffert, M.D. (Glaxo, Inc., 1987). A helpful patient-education resource available *free* through your physician or through Allen & Hanburys division of Glaxo, Inc., 5 Moore Drive, Research Triangle Park, NC 27709. (Ask for publication No. VIN 300.) Free.

Food Allergies

Food Allergy Publications

The Allergy Cookbook: Diets Unlimited for Limited Diets and *Allergy Cookbook for Festive Occasions* by Allergy Information Association, 65 Tromely Drive, Islington, Ontario M9B 5Y7.

Basics of Food Allergy by James Breneman, M.D. (Charles C. Thomas, 1984). An excellent text for physicians on food allergy. Charles C. Thomas Publisher, 2600 S. First Street, Springfield, IL 62708-4709. $54.75.

Cooking for the Allergic Child by Judy Moyer (Moyer, 1987). With more than 300 recipes for the entire family. Order from Allergy Control Products, 89 Danbury Road, Ridgefield CT 06877. $15.95.

Cooking with Isomil Soy Protein Formula. Ross Laboratories, Division of Abbott Laboratories, USA, Columbus, OH 43216. Free.

Diet and Behaviors. A report by the American Council on Science and Health, July 1987. ACSH, 47 Maple Street, Summit, NJ 07901. $2.00.

Food Allergy: A Primer for People by S. Allen Bock, M.D. (Vantage Press, 1988). This well-documented and well-organized book provides an up-to-date guide to understanding food allergies. $8.95. Vantage Press, Inc., 516 West 34th Street, New York, NY 10001.

Hidden Food Allergies by Stephen Astor, M.D. (Avery Publishing Group, Garden City Park, NY, 1988) Great resource. $7.95.

High Altitude Food Preparation. Colorado State University Extension Service. Pamphlet 530A. Wheat-, Gluten-, egg- and milk-free recipes for use at high altitudes and at sea level. CSU Extension Service. CSU Bulletin Room, Colorado State University, Fort Collins, CO 80523. $3.75.

Lactose Intolerance; Gluten Intolerance; Food Sensitivity. Each published by the American Dietetic Association, 430 North Michigan Avenue, Chicago, IL 60611. $4.75 each.

Meals Without Milk (1987). Mead Johnson, 2404 West Pennsylvania Street, Evansville, IN 47721. Free.

Newsletters

Because changes in subscription rates to newsletters are often difficult to predict, the prices of the following newsletters have purposely been omitted. Please contact the newsletter editor directly for samples or prices.

Asthma and Allergy Advocate. American Academy of Allergy and Immunology, 611 East Wells Street, Milwaukee, WI 53202 (414-272-6071). Contact: Robyn Brown.

The Asthma Team Newsletter. A newsletter for and about kids who have asthma. Your kids will love it! Christmas Seal League, American Lung Association Affiliate, 2851 Bedford Avenue, Pittsburgh, PA 15219.

Asthma Today. Leo Leonidas, M.D., editor. *Asthma Today,* 412 State Street, Bangor, ME 04401. A very informative monthly newsletter.

Asthma Update. David C. Jamison, editor. Quarterly newsletter that provides readers with the latest information available from medical journals about asthma. *Asthma Update,* 123 Monticello Avenue, Annapolis, MD 21401.

MA Report. Nancy Sander, editor. "A support system in a newsletter," published by Mothers of Asthmatics, Inc. Practical and positive information for parents of children who have asthma. Monthly. Send a self-addressed stamped envelope for free sample. Mothers of Asthmatics, Inc., 10875 Main Street #210, Fairfax, VA 22030.

The Newsletter. Jane Zukin, editor. A quarterly publication providing current information and support to those who suffer with lactose intolerance. Commercial Writing Service, P.O. Box 3074, Iowa City, IA 52244.

Pediatrics for Parents. Richard J. Sagall, M.D., editor. Demystifies medicine and allows parents to become active and informed partners in their child's health care. *Pediatrics for Parents,* 176 Mount Hope Avenue, Bangor, ME 04401.

Rodale's Allergy Relief. Mike McGrath, editor. Monthly newsletter published by Rodale Press. One of the best resource publications; helpful hints and product reviews. Sample issue, $2.50. *Rodale's Allergy Relief,* 33 East Minor Street, Emmaus, PA 18049.

Videos

American Academy of Allergy and Immunology, Learning Resource Center, Attn: Donna Kaczmarek, 611 East Wells Street, Milwaukee, WI 53202 (414-272-6071).

The Bee's Knees. Deals with insect allergy reactions and their treatment.

Immunotherapy—Old-fashioned or Futuristic. Informs patients about the basics of immunotherapy, its method and results.

What Americans Should Know About Asthma. This video features the inspirational stories of Olympic Gold Medalist, Nancy Hogshead and former world record holder and three-time Olympian Jim Ryun and helps to dispel common misconceptions concerning asthma. The video is perfect for use in patient-education workshops or in a support group-type setting. The information provided is valuable and leaves you feeling good about what you have seen. The film is accompanied by excellent teacher materials and posters made possible as a public service by a grant from Allen & Hanburys division of Glaxo, Inc. Order through West Glen Films, 108 West Grand Avenue, Chicago, IL 60611.

A Visit to the Allergy Doctor. Answers many of the questions patients ask during their first visit to an allergist. It deals with basic testing and common syndromes.

Nancy Hogshead's Aerobics for Asthmatics. This video offers a bundle of patient education through demonstration. The initial patient-education portion of the video is very informative though not the type of thing you need to hear or watch more than twice. The remainder of the video consists of a gentle warm-up period followed by gradually more aerobic activity before gliding into the cool-down. We liked the video overall because it was informative, practical and versatile. It could be used in an adult and/or adolescent asthmatic support group setting or in the privacy of one's home. Available through Aerobics for Asthmatics, Inc., 10301 Georgia Avenue, #306, Silver Spring, MD 20902 (301-681-6055).

Asthma and Allergies in the School: The Importance of Cooperative Care. This twelve-minute video is accompanied by two special editions of *MA Report,* one directed to parents and the other directed to teachers. The newsletters facilitate communication between the two parties and the video demonstrates managing asthma easily and effectively in the schools. There are no actors in this video. A joint production of Mothers of Asthmatics, Inc., and Fisons Pharmaceuticals distributed in cooperation with the Asthma and Allergy Foundation of America through Modern Talking Picture Service, Inc., 5000 Park Street North, St. Petersburg, FL 33709 (813-541-5763). Videos and newsletters are available at no charge on a loan basis or for purchase for a fee of $20.

Products

Air Filters

Aller/Guard, Inc.
Fleming Place Office Park
1121 South West Gage Boulevard
Topeka, KS 66604
913-272-4486

Allergy Control Products
28 High Ridge Avenue
Ridgefield, CT 06877
800-422-3878

Allergy Supply Company
P.O. Box 419
Fairfax Station, VA 22039
703-323-1111
800-323-6744

Biotech Systems
P.O. Box 25380
Chicago, IL 60625
312-465-8020
800-621-5545

Enviracare
747 Bowman Avenue
Hagerstown, MD 21740
301-797-9700
800-638-7416

High Tech Filter Corporation of America
80 Myrtle Street
North Quincy, MA 02171
800-448-3249
617-328-7756

Summit Hill Laboratories
Navesink, NJ 07752
201-291-3600

Newtron Products
3874 Virginia Avenue
Cincinnati, OH 45227-0175
In Ohio: 513-561-7373
800-543-9149

Research Products Corporation
P.O. Box 1467
Madison, WI 53701-1467
800-356-9652

Sentinel Room Air Purifiers
Farr Company
Department A
2221 Park Place
El Segundo, CA 90245
213-772-5221

Allergy-Proofing Products

Aller/Guard, Inc.
Fleming Place Office Park
1121 South West Gage Boulevard
Topeka, KS 66604
913-272-4486
  Dustproof mattress encasings (send for sample) and other products.

Allergy Control Products
89 Danbury Road
P.O. Box 793
Ridgefield, CT 06877
800-422-DUST
Dustproof mattress encasings (request fabric sample), Vacu-Filt, Miele vacuum cleaners, room air cleaners, quality books and more.

Allergy Supply Company
P.O. Box 419
Fairfax Station, VA 22039
703-323-1111
800-323-6744
A variety of home health products including mattress encasings, humidifiers and a number of other asthma-related items. Send for free catalogue or call for information.

Biotech Systems
P.O. Box 25380
Chicago, IL 60625
312-465-8020
800-621-5545
Distributors of allergy, asthma and respiratory supplies. Call for free catalogue.

Environtrol Corporation
P.O. Box 31313
St. Louis, MO 63131
314-966-6686
800-423-1982

Peak Flow Meters

Assess Peak Flow Meter
Healthscan Products, Inc.
882 Pompton Avenue
Cedar Grove, NJ 07009
Clear plastic. Suggested retail price, $19.95.

Biotrine Peak Flow Meter
Asthma Alert Peak Flow Meter
52 Dragon Court
Woburn, MA 01801
617-935-8844
  This peak flow meter has a whistle in it. If the child can make the whistle blow, his lungs are functioning properly. If not, there is some degree of airway obstruction. This meter comes from the manufacturer with an excellent, informative instruction book.

Mini-Wright Peak Flow Meter
Clement Clarke, Inc.
6947 Americana Parkway
Reynoldsburg, OH 43068
614-866-1465
800-848-8923
  Source of the Mini-Wright Peak Flow Meter, an excellent self-management tool for monitoring lung function at home. Durable, easy to read, accurate. Provides early warning of an impending attack. Prices vary from $29.95 to $34.95. Other sources of the Mini-Wright Peak Flow Meter: see Mothers of Asthmatics, Inc., Dura Pharmaceuticals; Allergy Supply Company

Nebulizers

Pulmo-Aide
DeVilbiss Health Care Worldwide
P.O. Box 635
Somerset, PA 15501-0365
814-443-1331
800-433-1331
  The Pulmo-Aide compressor nebulizer is designed with children in mind. The manufacturer has recently added a compact, portable nebulizer compressor to its product line, which can be used with a battery, connected to the cigarette lighter in a car or plugged into an electrical outlet. Includes both nebulizer cup, tubing, mouthpiece and face mask for easy delivery of .5 ml aerosol/minute. Contact a distributor in your area or call Biotech Systems or Allergy Supply Company (addresses given above).

Dura Neb 2000
Dura Phamaceuticals, Inc.
P.O. Box 28331
San Diego, CA 92128
619-789-6840
800-231-3195

The Dura Neb 2000 portable nebulizer is self-contained, compact and lightweight. A must for outdoor enthusiasts, kids and parents on the go! The company also makes a compact self-contained nebulizer compressor that looks similar to a lunch box or a very small fishing-tackle box. You can also order nebulizer supplies, and the Mini-Wright Peak Flow meter from Dura. Dura Neb 2000 is also available through local medical supply companies.

There are also other nebulizer compressors made by other companies; however, our experience with these two companies has never been disappointing. Good products, strong warranties and great customer service.

Allergy Vacuums

Nilfisk Vacuum
Environtrol Corporation
P.O. Box 31313
St. Louis, MO 63131
314-966-6686
800-423-1982

This company distributes Nilfisk vacuums and also carries a large selection of allergy products and air filters.

Nilfisk GS-80, 90
Nilfisk of America, Inc.
300 Technology Drive
Malvern, PA 19355
215-647-6420
800-NILFISK

Call for more information about this allergy vacuum. Also see Environtrol.

Miele 234i
Miele Appliances, Inc.
22D World's Fair Drive
Somerset, NJ 08873
201-560-0899
800-843-7231
  See Allergy Control Products (address given above).

Vita-Vac
Vita-Mix Corporation
8615 Usher Road
Cleveland, OH 44138
216-235-4840
800-848-2649
  Call or write for more information about the Vita-Vac allergy
vacuum.

Spacers

AeroChamber
Forest Laboratories
150 East 58th St.
New York, NY 10155-0015
212-421-7850
  The AeroChamber spacer should be available in most pharmacies.
If you cannot obtain one locally, ask your pharmacist to order one
for you from his supplier or through Forest Laboratories.

InhalAid
Schering/Key Laboratories
Kenilworth, NJ 07033
  See Allergy Supply Company or Biotech Systems (addresses given
above).

InsprirEase
Schering/Key Laboratories
Kenilworth, NJ 07033
  See Allergy Supply Company or Biotech Systems (addresses given
above).

Food-Allergy Products

Ener-G Foods, Inc.
P.O. Box 24723
Seattle, WA 98124-0723
800-331-5222

Vacuum-packed bakery breads, cookies, cakes, hamburger buns, doughnuts, and baking mixes with no wheat, eggs, milk and soy. Computer recipe service available to select recipes that comply with any dietary criteria. Some health food stores carry their products.

Miscellaneous

Acculevel
Syntex Medical Diagnostics
Palo Alto, CA 94304
800-528-5655
In California: 800-228-8244

The only finger stick blood test for theophylline! Your doctor can perform this test in his office and know the results in twenty minutes.

VentEase
Allen & Hanburys Division of Glaxo, Inc.
Research Triangle Park, NC 27709

The VentEase is a nifty little gadget that fits over the plastic sleeve of Ventolin and Beclovent inhalers. A local Allen & Hanburys representative should have ample stock on hand. Free through your physician.

"Tips for a Cleaner Burn"
Department of Environmental Quality
Air Quality Division
811 South West 6th Avenue
Portland, OR 97204

"Tips For a Cleaner Burn" is a consumer booklet about using wood stoves and alternative heat sources.

Quantum Eye
Quantum Group, Inc.
Sales Department
11211 Sorrento Valley Road, Suite C
San Diego, CA 92121
619-457-3048
800-824-9029
   The Quantum Eye measures the carbon monoxide levels in your home. Send a check for $10 for each CD detector you want.

Save a Life Allergy Kit
Karin Eisenhaure
265 Gilman Hill Road
RFD Mason
Brookline, NH 03033
613-878-2675
   Creative sack holds emergency meds on your belt. $5.50.

Sulfitest
Center Laboratories
35 Channel Drive
Port Washington, NY 11050

Support Groups

The Allentown Asthma and Allergy Support Group
Anne Keeler, President
923 Turner Street
Emmaus, PA 18049

Annapolis Hospital
Deborah Watson, R.R.T.
33155 Annapolis Street
P.O. Box 806
Wayne, MI 48184
313-467-4000

Asthma and Allergy Support Group of Arlington, Va.
Catherine Nnoka

1750 North Troy Street #694
Arlington, VA 22201
703-524-3168
703-857-1830

Ellen Metzgar, R.N.
Saint Mary's Health Services
200 Jefferson Avenue, S.E.
Grand Rapids, MI 49503
616-774-6738
616-774-6175

Sue Rutkowski
State Coordinator
Cooperative Care Program
33981 Spring Valley
Westland, MI 48185

Karen Bauer
AAF Regional Coordinator, MI
3620 North River Road
Freeland, MI 48623
517-781-2266

Florida State Chapter
Asthma and Allergy Foundation of America
1402 Dee Ann Drive
Brandon, FL 33511
813-684-3663
   Contact Kay Neville for unit information. This is a very active
group. For a complete listing of active Asthma and Allergy Foundation of America chapters and support groups, contact the Asthma
and Allergy Foundation of America (See Organizations).

St. Mary's Hospital Medical Center
1726 Shawano Avenue
Green Bay, WI 54303
Kay Tupala, R.N., Pediatrics Department Manager for St. Mary's
Hospital Medical Center
414-498-4200

New York Support Group for Parents of Asthmatic and Allergic
  Children
Caren Sanger
201 East 28th Street
New York, NY 10016
212-889-3507
   There are three regional groups which meet independently in
Manhattan, Queens and Westchester. Each group has a physician
adviser and meets once a month.

Parents of Asthmatic/Allergic Children, Inc.
Nancy Carol Sanker
1412 Miramont Drive
Fort Collins, CO 80524
303-482-7395
   A very active support group. Nancy Carol Sanker is also the author of a support group manual published by Mothers of Asthmatics, Inc., and is the contact for their Support Group Resource Council.

Parents of Asthmatic Children
Mary Sheridan
1 Freeman Avenue
Denville, NJ 07834
201-627-6875

Parents of Asthmatic Children
Greater Portland Area
Rae Brown
6 Poplar Ridge Heights
Falmouth, ME 04105
207-797-9188

Parents of Children with Asthma
Pam Greenman, R.N.
9450 Preston Trail East
Ponte Vedra, FL 32082
904-285-5680 (Pam—home)
904-358-3362 (Pam—office)

This group focuses primarily on infant to preschool children with asthma; however, all families are welcome. Meetings are held on the second Sunday of each month at 6:30 P.M. Call for location of next meeting.

Sequoia Hospital District
Linda Anderson, R.N., M.N.
Asthma Rehabilitation Coordinator
Whipple and Alameda
Redwood City, CA 94062
415-369-5811
Support group for adults with asthma and for parents of children with asthma. Meets on the second Thursday of every month. There is also an educational program for adults with asthma, nine sessions. Airpower program for children nine to thirteen and their parents. (Linda also notes that the local Lung Association has a support group for parents and kids with asthma. Contact Margo Leathers for ALA information at 408-998-5864.)

Vermont Lung Association
Janet Frances
30 Farrell Street
South Burlington, VT 05403
802-863-6817

Organizations

Most of the following organizations offer asthma and allergy information publications, networking or other helpful service. Write each organization for current information regarding services.

Allergy Information Association
65 Tromley Drive
Etobicoke, Ontario
M9B 5Y7 Canada
416-244-8585

American Academy of Allergy and Immunology
611 East Wells Street

Milwaukee, WI 53202
414-272-6071
1-800-822-ASMA

American Academy of Pediatrics
141 Northwest Point Boulevard
Elk Grove Village, IL 60009
312-228-5005

American Association for Clinical Immunology and Allergy
P.O. Box 912
Omaha, NE 68101

American College of Allergy and Immunology
Executive Offices
800 East Northwest Highway, Suite 1080
Palatine, IL 60067
312-359-2800

American Lung Association (New York Lung Association)
432 Park Avenue South, 8th Floor
New York, NY 10016
212-889-3370
   Chapters of ALA are nationwide; to find the chapter nearest you, look up American Lung Association in the phone book.

American Society of Internal Medicine
2550 M Street N.W.
Washington, DC 20037
202-289-1700

The Association for the Care of Children's Health
3615 Wisconsin Avenue N.W.
Washington, D.C. 20016
202-244-1801

Asthma and Allergy Foundation of America
1717 Massachusetts Avenue N.W., Suite 305
Washington, D.C. 20036
202-265-0265

The Center for Interdisciplinary Research on Immunologic
  Diseases (CIRID)
Georgetown University School of Medicine
3900 Reservoir Road, N.W.
Washington, DC 20007
202-687-1523
Contact: Virginia Taggart
  CIRID has developed programs for health care providers to use
with asthmatic patients. A program has been designed for the emergency room and booklets are available for physicians to be given to
both children with asthma and their parents. The materials are offered for a nominal charge to cover the cost of printing.

Mothers of Asthmatics, Inc.
Nancy Sander, President
10875 Main Street #210
Fairfax, VA 22030
703-385-4403

National Foundation for Asthma
Tucson Medical Center
P.O. Box 30069
Tucson, AZ 85751-0069
602-323-6046

National Heart, Lung and Blood Institute
NIH Building 31, Room 4A21
9000 Rockville Pike
Bethesda, MD 20892
301-496-4236

National Institute of Allergy and Infectious Diseases
NIH Building 31, Room 7A32
9000 Rockville Pike
Bethesda, MD 20892
301-496-5717

National Jewish Center for Immunology and Respiratory
  Medicine

1400 Jackson Street
Denver, CO 80206
303-398-1079
Lung Line
800-222-LUNG

Medical Journals

Parents and patients may find the following medical journals a good resource for research; however, parents should remember that the information is directed to doctors. Please do not draw conclusions without exploring your findings with a qualified physician.

American Journal of Asthma and Allergies for Pediatricians
Slack Incorporated
6900 Grove Road
Thorofare, New Jersey 08086
Subscription for one year costs $55. Published quarterly.

Annals of Allergy
American College of Allergy and Immunology
800 East Northwest Highway, Suite 1080
Palatine, IL 60067
Official journal of the American College of Allergy and Immunology. Subscription is $58 for one year. Published monthly.

Journal of Allergy and Clinical Immunology
C. V. Mosby Co.
11830 Westline Industrial Drive
St. Louis, MO 63146
Official journal of the American Academy of Allergy and Immunology. Subscription is $47.50 for one year. Published monthly.

Pediatric Asthma, Allergy and Immunology
Editor: Herbert Mansmann, Jr., M.D.
1651 Third Avenue
New York, New York 10128
Subscription is $90 for one year in the USA and possessions. Elsewhere: $123. Published quarterly.

Treatment Centers and Hospitals

Asthmatic Children's Foundation of New York
P.O. Box 568 Spring Valley Road
Ossining, NY 10562
914-762-2100

The Center for Allergy-Asthma-Immunology
Humana Hospital
20900 Biscayne Boulevard
Miami, FL 33180
305-932-0250

Children's Rehabilitation Hospital
3955 Conshohocken Avenue
Philadelphia, PA 19131
215-877-7708

National Jewish Center for Immunology and Respiratory
  Medicine
1400 Jackson Street
Denver, CO 80206
Lung Line
800-222-LUNG
303-388-4461

Asthma and Allergic Disease Centers

Duke University
P.O. Box 2893
Durham, NC 27710
919-684-5194
919-684-2922

Harvard Medical School
75 Francis Street
Boston, MA 02115
617-731-2129

Medical College of Wisconsin
Department of Medicine
8700 West Wisconsin Avenue
Box 12
Milwaukee, WI 53226
608-262-6954

National Institutes of Health
National Institute of Allergy and Infectious Diseases
Building 10, Room 11N250
Bethesda, MD 20205
301-496-7104
301-496-9314

Northwestern University Medical School
303 East Chicago Avenue
Chicago, IL 60611
312-649-8205

Scripps Clinic and Research Foundation
10666 North Torrey Pines Road
La Jolla, CA 92037
714-455-9100

Tufts University School of Medicine
136 Harrison Avenue
Boston, MA 02111
617-956-6880

UCSD Medical Center
225 Dickinson Center
San Diego, CA 92130
619-294-5580

Tulane University School of Medicine
1700 Perdido Street
New Orleans, LA 70112
504-588-5578
504-588-5263

University of California at San Francisco
Department of Medicine
400 Parnassus Avenue
San Francisco, CA 94143
415-476-2138
415-476-4537

University of Iowa Hospitals
Department of Internal Medicine
Division of Allergy and Immunology
Iowa City, IA 52242
319-356-2117

University of Texas Health Science Center
Dermatology Division
5223 Harry Hynes Boulevard
Dallas, TX 75235
214-688-2145

Centers for Interdisciplinary Research on Immunologic Diseases

Dr. Joseph A. Bellanti
Georgetown University School of Medicine
3900 Reservoir Road, N.W.
Washington, D.C. 20007
202-687-8219

Dr. John L. Fahey
UCLA School of Medicine
Center for Health Sciences Building
Los Angeles, CA 90024
213-825-6568

Dr. John P. Leddy
University of Rochester School of Medicine and Dentistry
601 Elmwood Avenue
Rochester, NY 14642
716-275-2891

Dr. Phillip S. Norman
Johns Hopkins School of Medicine
Good Samaritan Hospital
5601 Loch Raven Boulevard
Baltimore, MD 21239
301-323-2200

Dr. Charles W. Parker
Washington University School of Medicine
660 South Euclid Avenue
St. Louis, MO 63110
314-454-2501

Dr. Fred Rosen
Children's Hospital Medical Center
300 Longwood Avenue
Boston, MA 02115
617-735-7601

Scholarships

Academic Excellence
  Since 1987, Fisons Corporation has been awarding seven one-year
scholarships to high school students who suffer from asthma, have
demonstrated academic excellence and are planning to attend college. The first grant is for $5,000, the second is for $2,500 and the
remaining five are for $1,000 each. Entry forms may be obtained
from the American Academy of Allergy and Immunology (see Organizations) or directly from Fisons Corporation, Mr. Michael Fox, 2
Preston Court, Bedford, MA 01730.

Asthma Athletes
  An annual athletic scholarship is available through the Asthma
and Allergy Foundation of America funded by Schering Laboratories. (See Organizations for the Asthma and Allergy Foundation.)

Asthma Camps

Camps often move or change from year to year. Consult the following (listed under Organizations in this appendix) for more information:

The American Academy of Allergy and Immunology
The American College of Allergy and Immunology
The American Lung Association
The Asthma and Allergy Foundation of America

INDEX

Acetaminophen, 26
Adrenaline, 83
AeroBid, 75, 88
Air ducts, cleaning of, 131–36
Air filters, 131–34, 272–73
Albuterol, 14, 93–94, 118
Allergists, 52
Allergy-control plans, 100–1, 198
Allergy-proofing products, 273–74
Allergy testing, 6, 100–1
  preparing child for, 101–3
Alternate morning steroids (AMS),
  88
"Alternative" treatments, 66
Alupent, 74, 81, 117
Aminophylline, 10
Anticholingerics, 90–91
Antihistamines, 28, 75, 92, 103
Aspergillus mold, 134
Aspirin, 26
Astemizole, 93
Asthma management plans, 26–29,
  32–33, 50, 71, 77–79
  See also specific age groups, i.e.
  Infants; Teenagers
Asthma physiology, 5–7, 19–23
Atopic dermatitis, 152
Atropine, 90, 118
Atrovent, 90, 118
Attention craved by asthmatic
  children, 187–88
Azmacort, 75, 88

Baby powder, 176
Baby-sitters, 172–75

Bathing, 190
Beclovent, 75, 88
Beconase, 75, 94
Bedroom-cleaning, 127–30, 198, 200
Bed sheets, changing of, 43–44
Behavior problems caused by
  medications, 212–15
Bellanti, Joseph, 11
Berger, Janice, 199–200
Beta-adrenergic bronchodilators,
  74, 90, 92–93
  basic information, 79, 81–83
Birthday parties with food-allergic
  children, 158–160
Books and journals, 265–70, 285
Breast milk, 177
Breathing exercises, 39, 184
Breathing machines. *See* Nebulizers
Brethaire, 74, 81, 117
Bronkometer, 81
Bromfed, 75
Brompheniramine, 75
Bronchitis, 145
Bronchoconstriction, 20–23
Bronchodilators. *See* Beta-
  adrenergic bronchodilators
Bronchoscopy, 104
Bronkosol, 117

Camping with family, 227–30
Carbon monoxide, 142–43, 146
Carlson, Susan, 184–85
Car travel, 176, 233
Cat allergy, 151
Catalytic converters, 145

Catapress, 142
Central vacuum systems, 140–41
Chihuahua dogs, 45–46
Child care, 171–75
Children with Asthma (Plaut), 116
Chlorpheniramine, 75
Church nurseries, 171–72
CI-949 (medication), 151
Cilia in the airway, 22
Claritin, 208
Climate and asthma, 44–45
Coaches, talking with, 223
Colds, 23
Cold weather, 185, 223, 239–40
Corticosteroids. *See* Steroids
Coughs, 30–31
Crisis management of asthma, 70–72
Cromolyn, 75, 118, 208
  basic information, 83–84
Cures for asthma, 39, 67

Dating, 196–97
Deaths from asthma, 46–47
Decongestants, 75
Degrees of asthma (mild to severe), 22–23
Diary-keeping by parents, 12, 32–35
Dimetapp, 75
Disease centers, 286–89
Divorce by parents, 248–52
Doctors, 50
  bad doctors, avoidance of, 64, 66–68
  changing to a new doctor, 54
  educating parents about asthma, 60–61
  finding right doctor, 55–64
  good doctors, characteristics of, 51
  knowledge about asthma, 54–55
  office visit checklist, 65
  parent-doctor relationship, 58–62
  peak flow meters, attitudes toward, 56–57, 110
  questions from parents about treatment, 53, 57–58

referrals for doctors, 51–52
  second opinions, 63
  specialists, 52–53
  treatment philosophies, 54
Drugs. *See* Medications
Dust Mites, 44, 128–29

Early warning signals (EWS), 26, 168, 178, 181
  common signals, 26–27
Economics of health care, 68–72
Eczema, 23, 152
Electrostatic filters, 131
Emergency-room treatment, 72
Epinephrine, 83
Exercise, 196
  coaches, talking with, 223
  cold-weather concerns, 223
  medication prior to, 219, 220
  peak flow meters used prior to, 111, 208–9
  physical education, 208–10
  sports participation, 219–24
Exercise-induced asthma, 222–24

Family life with asthma, 244–60
Fiberglass disposable filters, 131–32
Fingernail color, 107
Fluids, child's need for, 176–77
Food allergies, 5, 6–7, 152–60
  diets for, 152–55
  family camping and, 227–29
  multivitamin supplements, 154
  "safe" foods, identification of, 154–55
  summer camp and, 227
  symptoms of, 152
  testing for, 100–1, 152
  vacations and, 235–36
Food-allergy products, 278
Fowler, Joseph, 98

Gastritis, 13–14
Gastroenterologists, 53
Gastroesophageal reflux, 27–28
"Growing out" of asthma, 42–44, 165

Hay fever, 198
Head and neck surgeons, 52
Health maintenance organizations (HMO's), 69–70
Heating fuels, 134
HEPA filters, 131
Hirsch, S. R., 187–88
Hisminol, 208
Hitchcock, Craig, 134–35, 136
Hogshead, Nancy, 209
Homebound instruction, 217
Humidifiers, 146, 175

IgE production, control of, 95–96
Immunologists, 52, 53
Immunotherapy (shot therapy), 76, 94–95, 100–1, 151
Infants and toddlers, asthma management for, 163–78
　advice from family and friends, 164–65
　attacks in progress, signals of, 168–69
　breast milk, nursing with, 177
　child–care concerns, 171–75
　early warning signals, 168, 178
　environmental controls, 176
　equipment, 167, 175
　fluids for child, 176–77
　medications, 96, 170–71
　tips for parents, 175–78
　travel precautions, 176
　triggers, 169–70, 178
Inhalers, 81–82, 180, 195, 197–98
　basic information, 122
Insurance for medical expenses, 67, 68–72, 120
Intal, 75, 84, 118, 208
Isoetharine, 118

Jenkins, Gail, 259

Kaliner, Michael, 11, 39, 54–55
Ketotifen, 12–13, 93

Lampl, Kathy, 209
Lanier, Bob, 42, 99, 141–42

Learning disabilities caused by medications, 91–92, 212–15
Lip color, 107
Loratidine, 93
Lung capacity, 112, 209
Lung damage, 48–49
Lung-function cycle, 113–14

McCarthy, Mickey, 172–74
McGee, Cheryl, 5–6, 9, 10–11
McGrath, Mike, 140
MA Report, 15–18
Mattress and pillow encasings, 127–29, 181
MaxAir, 81
MedAlert bracelets, 184
Medication Plan form, 80
Medications, 73–76, 77–79
　for allergies, 151, 207–8
　amounts needed, determination of, 114–15
　dispensing medication, tips on, 96–99
　for infants and toddlers, 97, 170–71
　myths about, 91–92
　new medications, development of, 92–96
　parents' need to be educated about, 60–61
　parents' questions, 78–79
　for seven- to twelve-year-olds, 190
　side effects. *See* Medication side effects
　for teenagers, 196
　for three- to six-year-olds, 182–83
　time to administer, 78, 79, 81
　types of medications, 77–91
　vacations and, 238–40
Medication side effects, 8, 9–10, 77–78
　of anticholinergics, 90
　behavior problems, 212–15
　of beta-adrenergic bronchodilators, 79, 81–82
　of cromolyn, 83–84
　in infants and toddlers, 170–71

learning disabilities, 91–92, 212–15
of steroids, 88
of theophylline, 85–87
in three- to six-year-olds, 182–83
Medication study programs, 11–13
Mendoza, Guillermo, 112–16
Metaproterenol, 117
Miele allergy vacuum, 137–38
Mild asthma, 22, 29–32
Milk allergy, 154–57
Mother-child relationship as cause of asthma, 40–41
Mothers of Asthmatics, Inc., 15–18
Moving the family, 44–45
Mucus production during asthma attack, 22
Myths about asthma, 36–49, 91–92

Nasalcrom, 75, 84, 208
Nasal irrigation, 124–25
Nasal polyps, 23
"Natural way" to control asthma, 48–49
Nebulizers, 116–22
  accessories, 119–21
  cleaning of, 121–22
  for infants and toddlers, 167
  medications used with, 82–83, 117–18
  purchase of, 119–21
  for seven- to twelve-year-olds, 190
  sonic nebulizers, 119
  for three- to six-year-olds, 182–83
  types of, 117–18
  vacations, use during, 228, 233, 237, 241
Newsletters, 14–18, 269–70
Nighttime asthma attacks, 113–15
Nilfisk allergy vacuum, 139
Nurses in schools, 205, 206

Opticrom, 75, 84, 208
Organizations, 282–85
Orthodontists, 53
Otolaryngologists (OTOs), 13
Otorhinolaryngologists (OTOs), 52

Ozone, 131

Peak flow meters, 12, 108–16, 188
  doctors' attitudes toward, 56–57, 110
  exercise, use prior to, 111, 208–9
  information on, 111–13
  makers of, 274–75
  medication amounts, used to determine, 114–15
  method of using, 111
  purpose of, 108–10
  for three- to six-year-olds, 182
  types of, 116
Peak Performance (Mendoza), 112–13
Pediatricians, 52
Penicillium mold, 134
Pets, 146–50, 151
Phenylpropanolamine, 75
Physical education, 208–10
Physiology of asthma, 5–6, 19–23
Pill-swallowing, 96–99
Plane travel, 233–34, 238, 241
Plaut, Thomas, 116
Play groups, 185
Pneumothorax, 48–49
Pollen, 44
Postnasal drip, 28–29
Precipitators. *See* Triggers
Preschool, 185
Proventil, 74, 81, 118
Pseudoephedrine, 75
Psychological disorders as cause of asthma, 37–39
Psychological effects of asthma, 42
Pulmonologists, 52–53

Remission, asthma in, 42–43
Respiratory distress, 48–49
Rewards for children, 98, 102, 179–80, 197
Rhinitis, 28–29
Rosenthal, Richard, 151

Sandoz company, 16
Sanker, Nancy Carol, 158–60

Scherr, Merle S., 225
Scherrer, Debbie, 16–17, 29–32, 58–62, 112–16, 145–46, 214
Scholarships, 289
School-related concerns, 202–3
  allergies at school, 198, 207–8
  homebound instruction, 217
  keeping child at home, 210–12
  learning and behavior problems due to medication, 212–15
  making up missed work, 216–17
  nurses in schools, 205, 206
  physical education, 208–10
  start of school, preparing child for, 206–7
  teachers, talking with, 203–6, 208–9, 210
  volunteering by parents, 215–16
Scouting, 229–30
Seldane, 75, 92–93, 208
Seven- to twelve-year-olds, asthma management for, 185–88
  equipment, 188–89
  medications, 189
  self-management skills, 186, 189–90
  tips for parents, 190–91
Sex and drug concerns, 200
Shampooing, 190
Siblings of asthmatics, 247–48
Side effects. *See* Medication side effects
Simulated asthma attack, 20
Single-parenting the asthmatic child, 252–56
Sinus infections, 13, 23
Sinusitis, 28, 125
Skin problems, 5, 23, 151
Sleep-overs, 191
Slo-bid, 86
Sly, Michael, 11
Smoking by parents, 141–46
  asthmatic child, effect on, 141–46
  quitting smoking, 141–43
Soy allergy, 158
Spacers, 94, 180–81, 188–89, 277
  basic information, 123

Sports participation, 219–24
Steroids, 10, 12, 14, 75, 94
  basic information, 87–90
Stethoscopes, 167, 181, 188
  basic information, 106–8
Stress, parental, 166–67
Stress as cause of asthma, 39, 249–50
Strunk, Robert, 216
Stuffed animals, 176
Sudafed, 75
Sulfite allergy, 157
Summer camps, 224–27, 290
Support groups, 62, 279–82
Sweat tests, 104
Swimming, 223
Szefler, Stanley, 214–15

Tagamet, 103
Teachers, talking with, 203–6, 208–9, 210
Teenagers, asthma management for, 191–95
  bedroom-cleaning, 198, 200
  equipment, 195, 197–98
  medications, 195
  self-management skills, 196–97
  sex and drug concerns, 200
Teenage years, return of asthma during, 43–44
Terbutaline, 117
Terfenadine, 75, 92–93, 208
Theo-Dur, 86–87
Theophylline, 10, 14, 74
  basic information, 85–87
  learning and behavior, effects on, 86–87, 212–15
Theophylline-level test, 87
Thermometers, 124
Three- to six-year-olds, asthma management for, 178–85
  early warning signals, 181
  equipment, 180–81
  medications, 181–82
  self-management skills, 179, 182–83
  tips for parents, 183–85

triggers, 181
Thrush, 89, 123
Ting, Stanislaus, 156–57
Toddlers. *See* Infants and toddlers
Tornalate, 81
Tracheitis, 145
Transition to controlled asthma,
   difficulties of, 185–88
Traveling parents in asthmatic
   families, 255–56
Travel precautions, 176, 233–34
Treatment centers and hospitals,
   286
Triggers of asthma attacks, 24, 169–
   70, 181
   common triggers, 24–25

Ulcers, 13–14

Vacation planning, 231–43
   activities, 232–33
   backpacks for children, 239
   car travel, 233
   cold-weather concerns, 239–40
   destinations, familiarity with, 232
   emergency room locations,
     knowledge of, 240–41
   finances, 236
   food, 235–36
   length of vacation, 236
   lodging, 234–35

medical exams, 238–39
medications, 237–38
nebulizers, 228, 233, 234, 241
plane travel, 233–34, 236, 238
pretreatments, 240
rest periods, 240
strollers, 239
trips abroad, 241
Vacu-Filt, 141
Vacuums, allergy, 136–41, 276–77
Vancenase, 75, 94
Vanceril, 88
Vaporizers, 175
VentEase inhalers, 122
Ventolin, 74, 81, 94, 118
Videos, 17, 209–10, 270–72
Viral infections, 23
"Vitamite" beverage, 156–57
Vita-Vac allergy vacuum, 136–37

Water Pik, 124–25
Weinstein, Allan M., 20
White, Martha Vetter, 11–12, 15, 26,
   74, 82–83, 92–96, 214
Wolf, Stanley, 209
Wood and coal stoves, 145–46
Working parents of asthmatic
   children, 257–60

Zaditen, 12–13